Kink

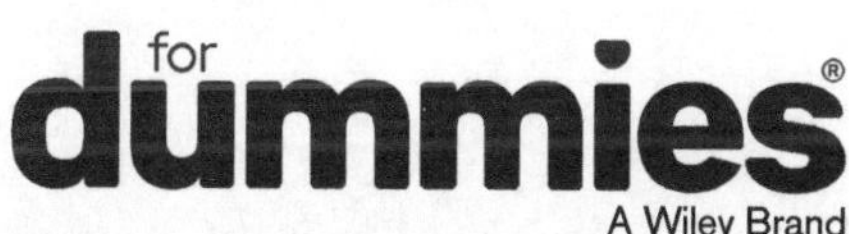

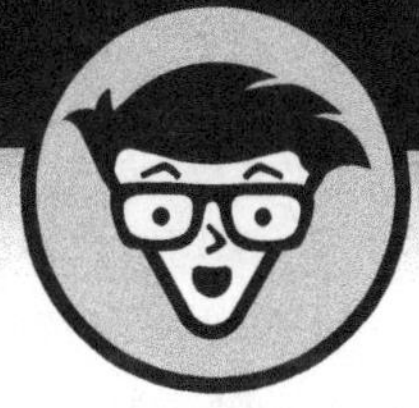

Kink

by Jaime M. Grant, PhD
with Jack Harrison-Quintana, MA

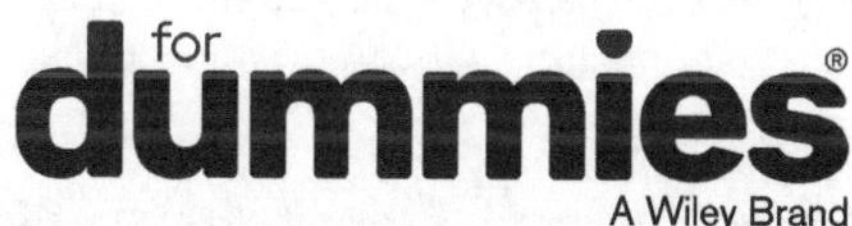

Kink For Dummies®

Contents at a Glance

Table of Contents

Introduction

hile kink is often portrayed as some kind of seedy, underground way of life, the truth is that there is a vibrant world of kinksters of all ages, races, genders, sexualities, and passions thriving all across the globe — in every culture, language, and religious and political environment.

Kink is common. Kink is intense! Kink is fun and *enlivening.*

And, it's been around for centuries. You can find evidence of kink relationships in ancient literature and art, and you can also decide to embrace kink in this moment. It's up to you to decide the meaning and place of kink in your life. We're assuming that's the journey you are on and why you picked up this book, and for certain — that's why we're writing it.

Because kink has been very meaningful in our lives for decades, we're excited to bring the experience of several of our kinky friends, loved ones, and colleagues to illuminate possibility for you. We hope to ease the path of discovery for anyone struggling with the swirl of tensions and contradictions that emerge when you consider pursuing your kinky desires.

Why does anyone engage in kink intimacy and connection given the widespread social stigma you are likely to encounter? What's the big attraction, and why would you take on that risk?

This book helps answer these core questions and hundreds more on a path to figuring out whether engaging in kink play — or drawing on kinky desire to build your most treasured, intimate relationships — is right for you.

About This Book

Kink For Dummies is for everyone on the journey to affirming and pursuing your deepest desires, even if they seem strange or perplexing. Kink longings often don't match up with the press-release or resume version of yourself, and that can be unsettling for kinksters at the outset of your kink exploration. Don't worry about this!

Upending your assumptions, dislodging your prejudices and fears, recreating your story of *you* as a desiring and desirable being — all of these are common steps in a kink discovery process. We're here for you, and so are 24 of our most brilliant and amazing collaborators, whose kink lives form a wild and woolly tapestry of passion, creativity, and commitment.

Together, we will address some of your big kink questions, such as:

>> What does it even mean to be kinky?

>> Is this desire that I want to pursue so much a kink?

>> How will I find others who want the things I want?

>> How do I talk to potential crushes or to my partner about this?

>> How do I make sense of this desire and fit it into the rest of my life?

>> What do I need to know to experiment, to try this out — safely?

>> How can I do this if I've survived abuse or violence in my life?

>> Who can I turn to for support?

>> Where can I find other kinksters and places to learn?

>> What do I need to think about to have kink desire and play be sustainable over the long haul?

>> How do I protect myself from the judgment of others?

We spend a lot of time in this book outlining practices of consent, safety, and care — not because kink involves widespread abuses, as is commonly charged. Actually, it's just the opposite.

Consent, safety, and care are cornerstone values in kink communities. By foregrounding and committing to expansive practices of consent, safety, and care, you literally have the room to try out the wildest and edgiest fantasies you can imagine. And you can do so within a community of people who are committed to ensuring that you have a safe and pleasurable experience.

Note: *Kink For Dummies* is a book about kink desire and relationships among consenting adults, and the ways they relate intimately and sexually. Many of the terms in this book clearly delineate sexual practices, experiences, and characteristics. Please proceed accordingly.

Foolish Assumptions

While writing this book, we made the following assumptions about you, dear reader:

>> You may be struggling or feel alone in your process of understanding and pursuing your desire, so we've written this book in the voice of an affirming companion for your journey.

>> You're curious but maybe daunted too. So, we've provided many self-reflective exercises and lists of tips and tools that will help guide your discovery process.

>> You're ready to reject any kind of fundamentalism or orthodoxy that keeps you from finding meaning in your life. Accordingly, you may need to turn down the volume from a lot of outside noise — even when it comes from people who love you.

>> You need more support. So we've provided multiple strategies and resources for finding like-minded explorers, experienced practitioners, new crushes, and future loved ones.

If there's one thing we hope you get from this book it's this: *you are the expert on you* — not us or anyone trying to sell you an off-the-shelf "fix" for your life. If we do our job right, you'll find a lot of accessible tools here so you can figure out what you really want, and how you want to build intimacy and relationships that matter.

Icons Used in This Book

This icon highlights information that deserves special attention.

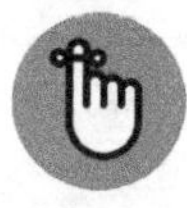

This icon gives you great ideas to consider and reinforces an important point.

This icon cautions you about bad thinking and roadblocks on your journey to self-discovery.

This icon introduces an interactive exercise that can help you figure out what your needs, values, desires, and next steps may be.

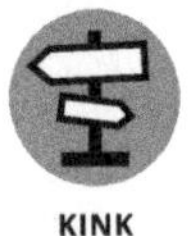

This icon introduces a personal story or example from one of the experienced kink contributors in our network of sex educators, activists, and kink enthusiasts.

Beyond This Book

Kink For Dummies is full of easy-to-digest information, analysis, self-reflection exercises, and resources about kink. But there's even more information available online! Just go to www.dummies.com and search for "Kink For Dummies Cheat Sheet" for additional support on your journey.

Where to Go from Here

If you're completely new to all of this, *Welcome!* We're so excited for you! This book is written for beginners, so just start with the first part of the book and find context, definitions, core ideas, and reflection exercises. These chapters cover so much ground, even seasoned kinksters will find new insights and helpful tips. If you get confused by any terms, go to the Glossary (see Appendix A) at the back of the book for help.

If you're already exploring kink, use the Table of Contents or index to find the topics you really want to know more about. Appendix B has some additional references, websites, and places to go from here. Get help on the issues that matter the most to you right now as you create an intimate life that is meaningful to you.

Remember to breathe. Thinking about kink desire and kinky play can go against a lot of foundational ideas in families and religious traditions. It can draw big reactions from your friends, lovers, or partners. But give yourself a break!

It's okay to question things — even *big,* fundamental things. It's okay to be curious and to seek information, supportive conversation, and resources as you figure out how to pursue lust, connection, and meaning in your life.

1

Getting Started with Kink Basics

Chapter 1

Introducing . . . Kink!

How to give kink an introduction worthy of its charms?

For some, kinky play offers a nearly spiritual portal to ecstatic joy; for others, it's a space to unleash your most degenerate, debauched self; and for still others, kink provides a place to release grief, heal, and build intimacy. Kink can be all of these things at different times, and more.

The purpose of this book is to help you discover what kink can be for you. It's chock-full of self-reflective exercises, checklists, assessments, tips, definitions, and even some great kink history. This mix of tools and stories should help you consider why your curiosity made you pick up this book, and what kinky experiments you may want to try. Here's a simple breakdown of the book so you can see what may be most useful to you on your kink discovery path.

Encountering Kink

The first part of *Kink For Dummies* will answer many of your basic questions. What do people mean when they say they are a Dom? What is a "praise kink"? Do Leather people actually wear leather all the time? What gives?

There are endless kink terms and practices to discover in the first four chapters of the book. You can just wander through these definitions and descriptions, or you can use them as a jumping-off point for deeper discovery. Take it all in, but don't think of it as the final word.

TIP

The magic of kink life is that new practices, new scenes, and new terminologies are constantly emerging.

One year a great film about tickling comes out and the community is awash in ticklers; the next, pup-play nights take over popular Leather bars and a million more kinksters are sporting pup hoods at events (see Chapter 4). This is the expansive and malleable nature of kink.

Creating Your Kinky Life

In Part 2 of this book, you can start to determine what kink means to you, personally, and what communication and relational skills you may need to develop to enjoy your kink desires.

In Chapter 6, for example, you'll get help addressing common questions: How do I reconcile my values for equality and respect with my desire to hurt or be hurt by my partners? How do I separate (or integrate) my identity at work or at home, with this person I want to become in kinky scenes?

I WISH I HAD SLOWED DOWN A BIT

For my start in kink, I would like to have spent more time listening to my body and really learning about the stoplight system (see Chapter 8) and making sure that I had greater degrees of trust with the people that I was exploring with. I realized that going slow is important, and that the concept that taking more pain makes you a better masochist is absolutely false. I've gotten past not wanting to disappoint people, now feeling connected with my own needs and directly expressing my boundaries. If I had a do-over, I would have liked to slow down my exploration at large.

Along my journey, I learned that you can use tools like spreadsheets to make things structured and clear! I was relieved to learn that you can have a spreadsheet for anything you want to try. There is so much ambiguity around what different roles can entail, and I wish I had given myself the space to learn in a more structured way earlier on. **—Gina**

And then, in Chapter 7, you can analyze your strengths and weaknesses as a communicator and think through what new skills you may want to develop. Co-creating consent and kinky scenes are discussed in Chapter 8, which includes a detailed checklist so you can explore your wildest fantasies inside a safe(r) container of your own making.

Dealing with Challenges

In Chapters 10 through 12, you can find very specific resources and ideas from our experienced kink contributors about how to manage emotional vulnerability and navigate common relationship challenges like jealousy and conflicting desires in your partnerships. If you are a trauma survivor, there's a whole chapter dedicated to sifting through what you may need to explore kink safely and get what you want. All relationships are work. And in kink scenes and relationships, the stakes are high to communicate well and care for your partners because some of the activities you engage in involve heightened emotional and physical risks.

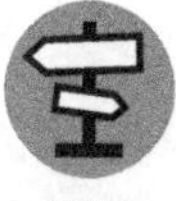

I think my superpower as a kinkster is that I keep letting people know when I'm struggling. I keep asking for help. I keep saying what I don't know. I use my safewords. I tap out when I'm overwhelmed. So, it feels like my kink life keeps expanding. It's a lot to juggle. But I'm always growing. I'm always learning more. **—Anonymous**

Playing for Keeps: Kinky Longevity

If you are fortunate to have a long-term relationship with kink, you'll go through many changes. You'll have to decide what social spaces align best with your kink temperament and needs. You'll have to navigate how public or private you want to be in your kink life. The kinds of kink you desire and pursue will likely morph and change over decades. What your body is capable of enacting will change. The meaning of kink intimacy with your partner or partners will grow, stretch, or contract with all of the life events that you go through together. In Part 4 of the book, you can look at how the unfolding of your life and your kink needs line up and diverge.

Finding Quick Reference Points

The chapters in Part 5 offer some great quick references for your kink journey, including rich insights and information at a glance. We answer questions like, what are the foundations of a great scene? What does a vibrant kink sexuality or relationship look like for me? And lastly, who are some amazing kinksters in history and in the present?

Your best partner in kink discovery is your curious, adventurous self. Try to free yourself from judgment and fear. Find a discovery buddy — a friend or social group — to experiment with and confide in. See Chapter 13 on getting out there and Appendix B, which offers a lot of kink resources that can help you along the way.

OUR RELATIONSHIP IS OLD ENOUGH TO VOTE

Rox and I are coming up on our 18th anniversary. And I said, *Oh, does that mean our relationship gets the vote now?* Like is our relationship finally "adult" at 18? I was joking, but also, there has been a real trajectory, like babyhood into adolescence into becoming more knowledgeable about ourselves and each other at the 18-year mark.

I think that there's a delicacy, especially when you're in long-term relationship with somebody around just recognizing that each other are human and that our bodies are sometimes not cooperative. And I think there's tenderness and beauty around giving each other grace around that and knowing that we change. **—Anna**

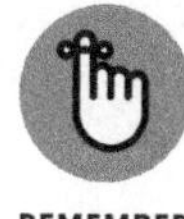

REMEMBER

Our bottom-line belief — the one that motivated us to write this book — is this: Everyone needs and deserves joy, intimacy, and connection.

Kink is an anarchic, unrestrained conductor of all of these. If you are here to figure out what kink might bring to your life, welcome to the journey.

Chapter **2**

Defining Kink

What does it mean to be kinky or to *have a kink*? By definition, a kink suggests there is a bend in the works, somewhere. When applied to your desire, having a kink means there's likely a twist to your sexuality — that somewhere in there, you want something that is seen as not traditional or customary. You can consider that to be your starting point.

There are seemingly endless variations in the ways *kinksters* (kinky people) live out their sexualities and their kink expression. In this chapter, we discuss the basics of kink so you can consider how your desires align with or depart from this intense world of intimacy and relationships.

Knowing Anything Can Be a Kink

A kink may be a desire that seems so far-fetched or different that you feel the need to hide, or sugar-coat, or even deny it among people you care about because you are afraid of what they might think. If you're worried you might be stigmatized or shunned at home, at work, or in your friend group because of how you want to connect intimately, it's likely that you have a kink.

But regardless of what others might think:

A kink is a desire or set of activities that have a magnified impact on you emotionally or sexually, propelling you into a heightened state of arousal and vulnerability. People often describe their first encounter with kink desire as overwhelming or consuming.

Beyond this basic idea of a kink as an enthralling quirk in the world of sex and pleasure, how do you distinguish your kinks from your other desires? And why are they so compelling?

Stepping into the kink universe

While many kinks have become widely known in popular culture — such as a desire to be tied up, or an urge to psychologically dominate a partner, others are much more obscure or undiscussed.

The following checklist of some common kinky desires that novices in the kink world might share with each other by way of introduction, or when attempting to discover whether your kinks are compatible.

KINK	DO IT TO ME	I WANT TO DO IT TO YOU
Make me follow your rules		
Gag me		
Yell at me		
Control my orgasms		
Handcuff me or tie me up		
Spank me		
Role-play with me		
Hurt and then comfort me		
Tickle me		
Play my Daddy or Mommy		
Keep me as your puppy or pet		
Call me names, humiliate me		
Worship my feet		
Force me to dress a certain way		
Blindfold me		

It doesn't matter if the compelling desire you've discovered is something other people know or talk about. What matters is that it's meaningful to you and might be something you want to explore with others. Chapter 5 takes you on a much more in-depth discovery process with your kinks.

Distinguishing between healthy and unhealthy desires

Take a breath. If you've been hiding a desire that is on this checklist, or maybe isn't on the checklist, but now feels possible to think about it — you may be activated. This means that your heart might be racing, and you might feel frozen, or a need to flee. Just breathe. It's okay to want what you want.

REMEMBER

The good news is, no matter how isolated you feel about your desires, there are people out there who share your kink interests. It's not the content of your kink that determines its value or propriety. It's what it means to you that matters (see Chapter 6).

Consent is the critical hinge that differentiates healthy kinks from problematic or damaging kink practices. For example, consensual pain may be mutually pursued and enjoyed among kink playmates and is the polar opposite of harm. Harm comes from having acts imposed upon you, your agency stolen, and your trust and your body violated.

In Chapter 3, we describe what consent and mutual respect look like in kink relationships, so you can figure out what you need to do or say in order to engage wholeheartedly and safely in any of your kink desires.

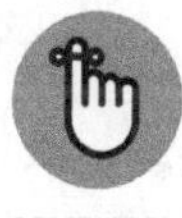

REMEMBER

The important thing to note is: *you are in charge.* You can enjoy any of the activities listed here — and literally hundreds of others not listed — in your mind, in your private fantasy life. This is a kink path that many people choose to create tremendous joy and pleasure in their lives.

DON'T YUCK MY YUM

An important value in kink communities is: *Don't yuck my yum.* If someone else's kink doesn't interest you — or seems disturbing — it's not for you. Move along. Find people who share *your* kinky interests and do what you love. But don't judge others for desires that seem peculiar or distasteful to you. Because the last thing you (or anyone) needs is that boomerang of judgment and disdain to fly back around at you.

Some people live full kinky lives on their own, in their fantasies. And if you decide that you want to take your kink desires out, beyond the confines of your imagination and your solo practices, into the world of kinky humans around you, there are all kinds of tips and resources to help you do this to your maximal delight and safety.

So, again, just breathe. You get to decide. No one else.

Connecting to formative experiences or unconscious shame

In decades past, kinky desires were often seen as wholly pathological. Kinky people — who we often refer to as *kinksters* — had to hide their desires and seek partners in various underground ways. Through word of mouth or community newsletters, people passed locations for kink cruising, bars where kink activities were supported, and community gathering spaces.

The problem with desires and communities that are suppressed or hidden is that they often pushed people into the realm of deep shame as they pursued romantic and sexual partners, and this left them vulnerable to predators who could blackmail or otherwise attempt to control them. All of this *forced a lot of harm onto kinky people* which then circulated in kink communities — further stigmatizing kink expression.

Suppression can also amp up the desire for a kink. Shame can contribute to compulsive thinking about kinks, and compulsive behaviors as well.

A very good reason to bring your kinks into the light, to name them and consider them in community, is to grow your self-esteem and your sexual and intimate health. There's nothing wrong with wanting to be intimate in ways that are out of the ordinary to some people. As long as you are not harming yourself, and are showing respect and care to others, you can fantasize or do whatever you want.

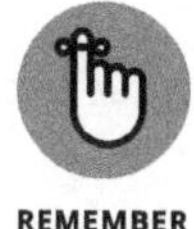

There's a world of difference between building your life in a state of shame and exploring how to play with feelings of shame in kinky space. The first is corrosive and endangering, and the second can be paradoxically liberating (much more on this in Chapter 6).

Today, kink is everywhere. You can find it in popular TV shows and on dating profiles in many dating apps. The very good news is that kink has come out of the shadows — there is a vast community of kinksters to find, and you can decide how open and visible you want to be as a kinky person.

And yet — there is still a lot of judgment out there.

You might decide to keep this part of your life private from extended family and coworkers (see Chapter 14 on Coming Out). Kink practices often call up and expose your most vulnerable self — and you can decide who, when, and how you want to bring people into this part of your life.

Excavating Your Kink Foundations

When Jaime was coming into her own kink expression, she kept wondering: Why are these desires so powerful? Why do they feel like nothing else in my life? Why am I so ashamed of them? In this section, you can start to explore these questions for yourself.

Giving yourself the space for discovery

Many of Jaime's coaching clients create a dedicated space for their kink explorations. We suggest you do the same as you make your way through the book. If you are struggling with shame or obsessive thinking around your kinks, a designated space can provide a container for you to open and close and might make this exploration and your experience of these desires more manageable. A digital file or old-school journal that you keep in a special drawer sends a message to your *struggling self. Like — oh, there's this safe space for all of these thoughts and wants. I can always come here when I need to, and I can also leave them here and go live my life.*

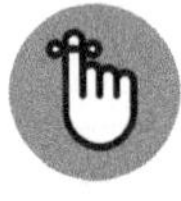

Creating a dedicated space for this work makes you the boss of this exercise, no one else. It can help you appreciate your own agency and personal power as you start to consider how you want to build your kinky connections and practices.

KINK DISCOVERY. Find a quiet private space for reflection. Get comfortable. Create an opening for you to discover more about your pleasure. In this exercise, let yourself revel in your kinky feelings and thoughts. Focus on a kink interaction that you fantasize about. Or you might want to center your thoughts on something you have read or a kink scene in a movie that has stayed on your mind. Answer these questions:

>> What is happening in your kink fantasies or in these situations you observed?

>> Who would *you* like to be in these scenarios?

>> What happens to you emotionally when you connect or observe someone connect this way?

>> What happens physically?

>> What parts of yourself come alive in your kink scenarios that are buried in the sexual or intimate life you are living?

>> How is this version of yourself different from the you that walks around in the world every day?

>> What might your life be like if you embraced these desires and allowed yourself the space to celebrate this version of yourself?

Write, write, write. Don't edit. Let yourself know more about your kinky feelings and potential. Let yourself stretch out into this part of yourself.

When you're done writing, close up your file or book and put it away. Return to it after you complete the Kink Detective exercise later in the chapter.

Over many years, Jaime has explored her kink desires through answering similar questions (because *geeking out* is one of her kinks; see Appendix A). She has been able to satisfy her curiosities about the role and meaning of kink in her life.

Many people have kink desires that are fantasies or practices that originate in profound formative relationships and experiences in their own lives. They also often connect to present-day pressures and constraints. Sometimes Jaime can draw a direct line from her kink to that experience — like the idealization of an authority figure in her childhood — and sometimes not. In the nearby sidebar, for example, Naria talks about the origins of her identification as a kink *Daddy* (see Appendix A).

Your kink desires may have formed as a response to the structures of social constraint and control around you in your family and society. For some people, it's their church; for others, an overbearing parent, partner, or boss. Kink expression is your way of surviving these pressures and pushing back on them, or insisting on yourself.

MAYBE I *SHOULD* BE YOUR DADDY

At a play party once, I had vice grips on my play partner Sara's nipples, pulling her toward me. She moaned, "Oh, Daddy . . ." and I was caught completely off-guard. My body knew something before my mind caught up.

"But I'm not your Daddy," I teased, somewhere between amused and surprised. Sara leaned in and said: "Well, maybe you should be . . ."

It was like someone flipped a switch inside me. The moment hit like a bolt of lightning, my whole body vibrating with the force of it. Everything I thought I knew about myself rearranged in an instant. I was a Daddy. And it felt like coming home.

For me, being a Daddy was never just about power dynamics or play — it was an extension of something deeply personal. My Daddy persona became an homage to the greatest man I've ever known: my father.

My Dad was the kind of man people gravitated toward. Sweet, kind, affectionate, and devoted to his family. He had a wicked sense of humor, progressive politics, and was the first male Feminist I ever met — long before the word was widely used. He and my mom shared a love that was passionate, playful, equal, and deeply respectful. He was my hero, my anchor, my role model.

A couple of days before my dad passed, he gave me a gift I will cherish forever. He and my mom had always supported my *BDSM* (see Chapter 4) identity and my activism in the Leather community, and in those final days, he looked at me with that familiar twinkle in his eye and said:

"You're a very good Daddy — to your wife, your partner, and to your son. I see how your family and friends love, respect, and trust you."

I carry those words with me every single day. **—Naria**

Sometimes the way that push-back forms seems logical — like, *I'm tired of being pushed around by bullies, so I want to play at being a dominant or a "bully" in my kink life.* Another common avenue for a bullying kink to develop may be — *I observed another person being bullied in a movie or on the playground when I was young, and I became surprisingly aroused thinking of myself as the bully, and it stuck.*

Sometimes, the opposite happens, and you may find that you've developed a kink that centers on your internalized vulnerability of being bullied, and you want to find a partner who will — *lovingly and carefully* — play at bullying you, in the manner you endured as a child, or saw in that movie, or are even experiencing in the present — perhaps at work.

Some kinksters will find themselves flipping back and forth between these two polarized roles, absorbing their exposure to bullying, and the erotic charge it created, by developing a flexible or versatile kink embodiment of the bully over time.

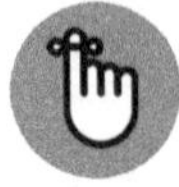

Transformative re-enactments are a staple of kinky life.

REMEMBER So many people have survived a vast array of harms — from being bullied as in the previous scenario, to being assaulted physically or sexually; displaced from home due to war or economic distress; humiliated by authoritarian control by a boss or the police; marginalized due to neurodivergence or mental illness; or shunned by family members or peers.

Kink expression can be a vehicle for working through devastating experiences by turning them on their head, transforming the echoes or remnants of harm into a source of pleasure and connection.

TIP

This is where some of the controversy around kink arises, and why for years mainstream psychological theory cast all kink expression as pathological. Like many early psychological theories — such as women are "too emotional to be leaders" or LGBTQ+ people "are sick" — kink pathologization has been widely discredited, and many psychologists now understand kink practices as offering underappreciated, creative paths to vibrant intimate connection and healing. You can explore more about this in Chapter 11.

I SAW THE BAG OUT OF THE CORNER OF MY EYE

At a Leather festival, I once saw a Dom put their sub into a black leather full-body restraint device that many people refer to as a "sleep sack" but I call a *body bag.*

I felt an immediate pull, but it wasn't until a decade later that my desire to buy one hit its peak. At that time, the amount of responsibility I was carrying in my professional life had spiked, and along with that came an increased desire for me to give up control in my sex life.

I had a friend with an experienced Dom partner who I played with. Sometimes he would spank me or slap me around, and then after we both orgasmed, he would play ambient music, put me in the body bag, and then leave me alone in the room with the lights off for an unspecified amount of time he would determine without informing me.

It was the best feeling. Not having any option to do anything other than breathe and relax allowed me to *let go* at a level I had never been able to achieve before. I live with chronic anxiety that I treat with a daily medication that really helps, but still leaves me with higher-than-average anxiety.

One thing I know being restrained does for me is that it keeps me off my phone. I check it all day long and sometimes it serves up something that connects me to my hobbies and my joy. But I never know when it might also bring a professional e-mail that spikes my anxiety. When I first bought the body bag, I was receiving e-mails all day and night from people above me in the hierarchy of the company who expected swift and thorough responses, regardless of whether it was during normal working hours. My Dom and the body bag freed me from all of that. **—Jack**

You may or may not know — or want to know — where your kinks come from. That's okay. You don't need to know. All you have to do is figure out whether pursuing kinky connection is something you want or need to feel true to yourself in your intimate life. And, as you read this book, we hope you come to understand that whatever your kink, you're not alone. Many others have fixated or settled on the specific kink desire that you may be interested in. It's possible to find community and partners, if that is what you want to do.

I SHOULDN'T WANT WHAT I WANT

As a feminist, for many years I denied my kinky desires for submission. I had been disowned as a young person for being a lesbian — out on my own in my early 20s, always in charge at work, living solo, determined to make my way. I longed for some place to give up control and to have someone else take over and take care of me. But I thought this was wrong, a sign of weakness or internalized sexism. And then I found a few incredibly attentive lovers who let me share this vulnerable side of myself. And I discovered that my fears had just been unfounded. Instead of disrespecting me,

(continued)

(continued)

> these partners accepted my submission as a sacred gift. They treasured me, in and out of the bedroom. And while I had worried that pursuing these desires might disassemble me psychologically, it turned out that submitting in bed gave me more strength in my daily life. I was actually better at standing up for myself in my friendships, my family of origin, and at work. **—Jaime**

Many people enjoy their kinks without thinking too deeply about where they come from or what they mean. But in Jaime's coaching practice, she finds that many clients experience "not-knowing" or the un-excavated origins or meanings of their kinks to be a barrier to their pleasure and self-discovery. So in this book, we offer a lot of different activities for you to figure out as much about your kinks as you like.

ACTIVITY

KINK DETECTIVE. In this exercise, you can start to consider how your kink desires connect to your formative and ongoing experiences of enduring various pressures and constraints. You'll reflect on formative and present-day experiences that:

» Have an idealized person or quality to them.

» Have a possible shame component.

» Have or are constraining you, tearing you down, or making you feel ashamed or less-than.

Take notes, don't edit, and write knowing you never have to show these to anyone else.

IDEALIZATION DISCOVERY

Think about who you idealized as a child, and ask yourself the following questions:

» What were their characteristics?

» Do you remember an experience of interacting with them while they were being powerful or beautiful or overwhelmingly amazing?

» How did you feel around them?

» Did you want to become them?

» Did you want them to love you more?

» Did they love you the most and idolize you?

» Did they ignore or dismiss you?

Write about the atmosphere, feelings, sounds, and colors you associate with this idealization.

Similarly, do you have someone you idealized as a young adult or currently? (Or perhaps a book or movie character left a significant erotic imprint on you.) Ask yourself the following questions:

>> What are their characteristics?

>> Do you remember an experience of interacting with them while they were being powerful or beautiful or overwhelmingly amazing?

>> How did (or do) you feel around them?

>> Do you want to become them?

>> Did (or do) you want them to love or respect you more?

>> Do they love or respect you the most and idolize you?

>> Do they ignore or dismiss you?

Write about the atmosphere, feelings, sounds, and colors you associate with this idealization. Include who you get to become around this person.

FEAR, SHAME, OR HUMILIATION DISCOVERY

Think about a formative or young adult incident of fear, shame, or humiliation that has stayed with you. This may have involved the way someone related to you or involved seeing or reading something that caught your attention.

>> What were the characteristics of these people or this connection?

>> How did you feel when it happened?

>> Did you want to please the perpetrator in the scenario?

>> Did you want to harm them? Did you want them to love you more?

>> What kind of power did they have over you, and how did they wield it?

Remember what it was like during that time. Write about the atmosphere, feelings, sounds, and colors you associate with this fear or shaming situation. Write and put yourself back there.

When you finish your Kink Detective notetaking, pull out your Kink Discovery exercise earlier in this chapter and look at them side by side. Ask yourself:

>> How do these discovery processes fit together?

>> How do these exercises echo or call out to each other?

>> How do compelling formative experiences or your daily strains and stressors inform your kink desires or needs?

Write, write, write — and don't edit! This activity will help you understand more about your foundational kink nature and appreciate the specific pathways to your kink pleasures. Everything doesn't have to fit like a matchy-matchy suit. Look at atmospheric connections, search for tensions and contradictions in each situation. Examine your story for possible clues about your marvelous kinky potential.

Zeroing in on some kink truths

People who are new to kink can find themselves in a jumble of new ideas, and seemingly contradictory or confusing language. It can be hard to figure out standard ways to talk about or consider various ideas and possibilities. One reason for this is because kink worlds are so layered and complex, two people may experience the same set of kink experiences quite differently. One person's way of talking about a desire or way of being may be the opposite of another's.

This complexity may be confusing for you as you embark on your kink journey. Absorbing the vast field of kink play can be overwhelming and possibly lead you away from things you already know — from your own internal sense of self or your intuition.

For example, many people consider kink and sex to be the same thing, but many kinksters have a thriving kink life that involves great vulnerability and closeness with their play partners, but no sex — and by that, I mean, no touching of the genitals or other sexy body parts. A kinkster like this may say, *this is my play partner, but not my lover.*

And another kinkster might experience and talk about this quite differently. They, too, may have a play partner they are very intimate with and have no genital involvement, and may say: *this is my lover and my primary partner.*

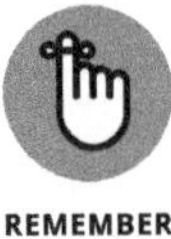

Play partners are not always lovers; lovers are not always play partners. You can have deep love, connection, vulnerability, and intimacy with a play partner who is not your lover, and a lover who is not your play partner.

REMEMBER

And yet another kinkster can live these very same conditions and say: my kink is my sexuality, or my sexual orientation *is kink.*

All of these kinksters are quite right, of course, because they are describing their own experiences (see Chapter 6 for more on how kinky people make meaning). A few important take-aways from this example of complexity for the kink beginner are:

>> **Don't assume.** Whatever your definitions of sex and kink are, they are meaningful to you. Don't assume they are meaningful or apply to others.

>> **Ask.** When you don't understand what another kinkster is telling you about their kink desires or their lives, don't impose your labels on their experience. Instead: Ask.

>> **Adopt a learning posture not a testing posture.** Kinksters are curious. You are stepping into an expansive community of people who defy categorization. The idea is not to create tests or imperatives for various identities and put people into boxes. Instead, be open to learning.

>> **Affirm, appreciate.** Kinksters are so ingenious and creative. They have often persisted in their discoveries and inventiveness despite hardships, terrible judgments, and backlash. Always remember to affirm, appreciate, and enjoy!

Understanding what influences you

Kink is about taking up space socially, sexually, and intimately that the prevailing religious, cultural, and political systems would deny you; such as

If you're a hunky football player, you "shouldn't" want your partner to *peg* you (see Appendix A). If you're a pacifist, you "shouldn't" get hot watching brutal militarized sex scenes. If you're straight and largely traditional around sex, you "shouldn't" want to go to clubs to watch gay Dominants flog or otherwise exert power over their partners.

The kinksters in the previous scenarios are being resistant to pushing against the "rules" associated with their identities. However, kink is about claiming any and all unwieldy, "unacceptable" desires. It's about breaking out and breaking free.

We live in social and political worlds that are steeped in power relationships; often, someone is winning, while another is losing. One nation is exerting power, and another is submitting to it. A parent or teacher is setting all the terms of success for a child, and the child is doing their best to rise to expectations and survive the pressures in the system.

All of these are the formative "gasses" that shape us. They shape our conscious life and relationships, as they shape our unconscious life and our sexuality.

It makes perfect sense then, that our kink fantasies are a product of our survival in this demanding order of things. When seen through this prism, our kink desires are a brilliant, creative commitment to relationship, to our intimate life, and to our longing for connection in the face of a lot of alienating structures.

When we see our kink desires this way, we don't just love and appreciate all of the astonishingly beautiful experiences and people they've brought to us. We are proud and amazed by them.

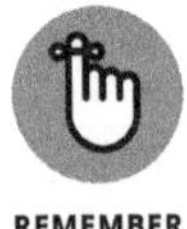

A paradox of kink is that while often grounded in an experience of overwhelm or shame, kink is a portal to ecstatic, joyful, expansive experiences and relationships. Or, shame and humiliation in our day-to-day lives are draining and unsexy; meeting your abject or intensely vulnerable self with a worthy intimate partner can be explosively sexy.

Chapter **3**

Grounding Kink in Consent

In this chapter you'll get all the information you need to construct responsive, fully consensual kinky practices. Consent is obviously crucial in kink situations, where your physical and emotional vulnerability is high, but building great consent practices will serve you in every area of your life.

Here, we present different ways to assess your level of self-knowledge around your kink desires. We also offer examples of transparency and mutual respect so you can consider how these are operating (or not) in your relationships and sexual life.

Realizing that Consent Is King

There is nothing that has generated more discussion in kink communities than practices of co-creating and exchanging the terms of consent. In the face of stigmatization and unwarranted charges of abuse by mainstream culture, kink communities grew an equally strong commitment to ensuring pleasure and community care. Ground-breaking consent conversations and practices emerged that have become a model for all people engaging in intimate relationships.

Knowing how to build consent — by drawing and redrawing healthy boundaries in your intimate life — creates health and vitality everywhere.

Digging into the history of kink and consent

In 1983, a member of a gay men's kink group in New York City, David Stein, coined the term *Safe, Sane, and Consensual* to describe the group's values and practices around kink encounters. This work had a reverberating impact in kink organizations, pushing back on the idea that kink relationships were inherently sick and abusive. For over a decade, Safe, Sane, and Consensual was the driver of consent practices in kink communities.

This framework ignited a lot of conversation about the elements of safety and physically and emotionally sound practices in crafting consent. For example, could play partners drink or drug and stay safe and sane? Could survivors of abuse play with scenarios that brought to mind their victimization, and take care of themselves emotionally? For many years, Safe, Sane, and Consensual helped people consider their personal limitations and also the environment in which kink play occurred.

Then in 1999, Gary Switch posted another term to a different major group's list-serv, the Eulenspiegel Society, *Risk Aware Consensual Kink* (RACK), noting that like any daily activity — say driving to work or taking a hike — all forms of kink expression involve risk, so that no matter how well planned, no kink interaction can ever guarantee perfect safety. Within the RACK framework, players are prompted to be responsible for their own well-being as they assess the capacities of each person in the mix.

RACK acknowledged the complexities of playing in emotionally and physically fraught arenas, noting that some *kinksters* (kinky people) experience regret in aftermath of a carefully orchestrated scene. This happens even when consent has been clearly mapped out. RACK noted that even when all people in a kink interaction prioritize the well-being of their partners, things can still go wrong, or end badly.

After RACK emerged, *Personal Responsibility, Informed Consensual Kink* (PRICK) followed soon after, which really zeroed in on the responsibility of the individual in kink reactions. Both RACK and PRICK emphasized that anyone in a kink scenario is responsible for themselves in assessing their vulnerabilities.

In the ensuing years, many other acronyms emerged; but significantly, in a 2014 article published in the *Electronic Journal of Human Sexuality*, DJ Williams, Jeremy N. Thomas, Emily E. Prior, and M. Candace Christensen swung the consent discussion back toward a more communal value of care: *Caring, Communication, Consent, and Caution* (CCCC). By foregrounding care, rather than personal awareness or responsibility, the authors suggested that care is a fundamental value in kink communities that drives connection, and the moment-by-moment adjustments made in any scene. Yes, each person is responsible for themselves in a kink interaction, but together, collectively, everyone in a kink environment is surviving a violent, anti-sex, inequitable culture. Accordingly, kink players should foreground attending to these inequities, by championing solidarity with each other, and taking on responsibility for well-being within a connected community. Care is then a shared value and a shared responsibility.

We offer this history to illuminate how seriously kinksters have wrestled with the question of consent over many decades. We have moved in many activist and social justice communities over the past 30 to 40 years, and Jaime ran a rape crisis center as a young person. And the level of engagement with ideas about consent and the passion and creativity kinksters have applied to the challenge of co-creating consent is quite remarkable and admirable.

In our humble view, kinksters have been true leaders in this work, innovating and improving consent practices far beyond the kink communities.

As you move into kink spaces, organizations, and communities, checking out how they talk about consent is an excellent way to consider which groups feel like the best fit for you.

WHY DO THEY CALL IT A SCENE?

Kinksters love to create *scenes* together. Like a scene in a play, everything is choreographed in advance. Perhaps there is even a detailed script. At the very least there is a *consent or scene container* for the kink action that details what can and cannot happen, and what activities are likely to bring immense pleasure to the actors. Also like the theater, people in the scene are taking on roles that are not like those they inhabit at work or in everyday interactions. In many cases, they are quite the opposite. So over time, the language of "player" and "scene" evolved to note that kink interactions are distinct from the daily ways you interact. They're elevated or intensified — emotionally, socially and sexually.

Kink community practices around substance use and consent

Drinking alcohol and using other drugs creates an artificially induced altered state. Accordingly, drinking and drugging while engaging in kink play compromises your ability to report on your condition and assess your partner's physical and emotional state in a scene. Nonetheless, some kinksters choose to drink or drug when they play.

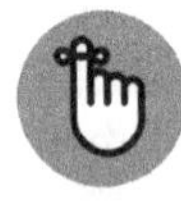

When your mind has expanded — by an endorphin rush or by an ingested substance — you're likely floating in a euphoric cloud of intimate joy or astonishment. Accordingly, what you want in that moment often does not reflect what you are emotionally or physically capable of.

One of the reasons kinksters have trailblazed the practice of fully outlining consent *before* a kinky interaction, is that it's widely understood that the altered state brought on by a kink-induced endorphin rush (*see* Appendix A) creates *heightened vulnerability*. Alcohol or drug induced altered states create a comparable or even greater vulnerability.

Many kink dungeons and play parties train safety attendants, sometimes called *Dungeon Monitors* to roam through the various scenes and keep an eye on the well-being of all the players. Their specific charge is to end play should a participant appear to be drunk or otherwise high. This practice is embedded in a larger set of values and practices around consent and community health.

Drugs and kink are not a good mix. Kink culture highly discourages and, in many cases, wholly prohibits kinky action while drinking or drugging. If you refer to community agreements at the vast majority of the established Leather and kink social clubs in the U.S. and around the world, drinking and drugging while engaging in kink play is either prohibited or highly discouraged.

SAMPLE SUBSTANCE USE POLICIES

Here are just a few sample substance use policies from kink social clubs:

NO ALCOHOL, FIREARMS or any ILLEGAL DRUGS may be brought into the dungeon. Anyone who is noticeably affected by either alcohol or drugs will be denied admittance.
—The Guild of Deviated Standards

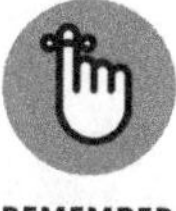

An enraging paradox in kink life is: While mainstream condemnation about kink play is that it's risky or endangering, that assessment often comes from non-kinky people who are having sex with little to no consent discussions, drunk or high, on a regular basis.

Building Consent: The Essentials

In kink life, consent is a constant conversation. Because kinky practices move you into tender and sometimes fraught or contradictory emotional territories, consenting to play in these spaces must be explicit and crystal clear. In her early days of doing consent education on college campuses, Jaime often noted the most important aspect of engaging in consent conversations:

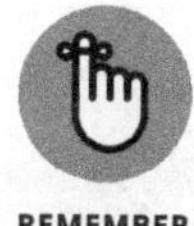

Consent is relational, not transactional. It isn't a one and done prospect in any intimate or sexual situation. Instead, it's an ever evolving, flowing exchange of feelings, body cues, and information.

Think of consent like partner dancing, although kinky play and sex are much more complex than, say, doing the foxtrot around a crowded ballroom. The core idea about the comparison is that you must constantly read and adjust to your dance partner.

A single "yes" before engaging in kink or sex doesn't mean you can do *anything* after receiving that answer. The days of monolithic or one-dimensional consent are long gone.

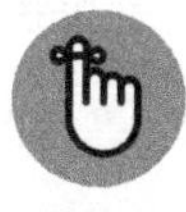

Reading body cues, communicating well, showing up with care, and articulating explicit limits are all a part of an excellent consent ballet for everyone involved.

Today, consent conversations rest on a three-legged stool of self-knowledge, mutual respect, and full disclosure or transparency. As you develop skills and understanding in these three key arenas, you build a strong foundation upon which to co-create flexible, dynamic and effective consent containers (see Chapter 8 for more information on creating a consent container). And, as CCCC suggests, you enter a community that values care and caution as you interact with potential players or lovers.

WE DON'T LIKE THE WORD *NEGOTIATION*

A big word in kink world and consent conversations is: *negotiation*. Kinksters often talk about negotiating a scene, by which they mean putting all of the participants' desires and limits on the table, so that together, you can build a kinky happening that is sexy, enlivening, and perhaps pushes everyone to their ecstatic limits.

But negotiation is a term most often used in business transactions. In a business negotiation, both people are trying to win, while one is often in a more vulnerable position, trying to hold onto the value of their labor or idea. Often, one person has an advantage, like more money, or ownership of a property that the other needs, and the other is struggling or compromising to get what they need so they can do what they really want to do.

In our mind, this is the opposite of what kinksters do in a co-created consent conversation. Instead, you are working with a partner to balance whatever is messed up in the system — for example, inequities that designate one of you as powerful and the other not; physical differences; anti-sex ideas about what is appropriate or available to you; *trauma burdens* (see Appendix A) — so that everyone is equally gratified by the outcome. In effect, you are all winners.

Our bottom-line needs in a scene are not up for negotiation, and yours shouldn't be either. Hence, instead of negotiation, throughout the book, we use the terms *co-creation* and *consent conversations*.

Knowing yourself

What does it mean to know yourself in a kink situation, especially if you are new to kink? How do you set limits when you don't even know what you like yet?

In Jaime's book *Great Sex: Mapping Your Desire*, she notes that the vast majority of her coaching clients — in any sexual situation — don't know what they want. Often, authority figures or formative experiences of shame have led them to bury their desires or present a kind of sexy false front that has little connection to who they are and what they really long for.

Accordingly, she offers several core questions to start the process of digging into your story for clues to how you want to connect in your intimate life.

DESIRE MAPPING. Try to answer all of the following questions. Don't edit yourself. You don't have to share this with anyone. You can do this exercise once, or over weeks or months or years.

Here are your starting points.

> » Have you left important parts of yourself behind on your path to forming your sexuality or the expression of your desires?
>
> » Have you been hiding a bit to be more presentable or to make things "easier" for your partners?

Because many of us develop our sexualities in coercive, dangerous, or risky situations, it can be hard to go back and sift out the things you learned about yourself as you were coming to understand your desires. Unfortunately, this often leads people to shut down and deny themselves, which is not a good foundation for figuring out your kinks and your limits.

If this describes you, don't worry. Many Desire Mapping clients have started from a shut down, frozen, or fake place in their desire discovery journey. Through desire mapping, they have come to a much more honest, enlivening path around their sexuality.

With the next set of questions, you can begin to claim the real you and grow your self-knowledge as you step into the world of kink.

> » What encounters or relationships stand out as most significant over the course of my sexual life?
>
> » What sexual experiences or experiences of my desire made me feel most true to myself? Why?
>
> » What specific sexual experiences or encounters with my desire have elicited the most intense physical and emotional responses in me? Why?
>
> » When did I learn something important about myself, even if it was something I never wanted to learn? What was it?
>
> » What lover(s) or crush(es) do I most miss and what do I miss about them?
>
> » What have I always wanted to do sexually, but have held myself back? Why? What stands out as a big, missed opportunity for me to explore my desire?

The information you are gathering in your Desire Mapping process can be a great way to begin consent conversations with a kink partner. An excellent kink partner will be thrilled to have these conversations with you.

And, most importantly, the following questions can help you start to apply what you're learning to build a more honest and vibrant intimate life.

>> Am I living out the desires I've found to be important to me in this exercise?

>> Am I denying or hiding my desire out of fear or judgment?

>> Do I have new information here that can help me inform kinky partners about what I want to explore?

>> How can I bring these discoveries into the creation of the kinky life I imagine?

As you grow your store of knowledge and inner conversation about your desire, you may want to bring others into this process to help you reflect and support your exploration. Many Desire Mapping clients take their desire maps to their friends or therapists or support groups. Chapter 13 provides a lot of information about how to build community and resources as you grow your self-awareness and experiment with kink connections.

Defining consent agreements

Along with self-knowledge, understanding the basics around mutual respect and balancing power are core competencies in kink life. In this section, we discuss how consent practices involve the co-creation of agreements among equals, requiring full disclosure (or transparency) and mutual respect. When these three elements are present, you can rest assured that you are taking the best care of yourself and your partner(s) as you venture into kinky territories that may seem especially vulnerable or risky.

Consent among equals

We'll spend a fair bit of ink in this book on the concept of safety in your kinky life and practices (see Chapter 4). This is not because kink is inherently problematic or unsafe as its detractors suggest. Rather, kinky connections can often bring you into euphoric states of being where you want to do more, go farther, or try yet another activity you've been fantasizing about. And that's one of the true wonders of kink — the expansive possibilities it can create.

But taking care of yourself in that space is an extra bit of work.

Agreeing in advance about what your limits are and where the line is around experimentation can be especially important because — speaking specifically for ourselves and our many loved ones in the kink world — it can be so easy to get carried away in the cloud of lust and adoration you have for a partner. You can forget about the limitations of your body or your psyche. You can just want *more*. Accordingly, we take extra care when we find a partner who can open the door to these ecstatic states of being, and we want you to do the same.

Consent among equals is a complex idea. You can see the evidence of gains in the fight for equality in kink organizations and communities:

>> BIPOC and LGBTQ+ people, and women across various identities are writing books and producing kink podcasts, leading the conversation and consent and equitable practices.

>> These kink experts and communities are centering their needs in kink spaces, helping kink communities think critically about balancing power, especially when referencing anti-queer, sexist, or racist tropes in kink play (more on this in Chapter 4).

>> Legal gains around housing and employment equity mean that people who have typically been vulnerable in relationships are often experiencing less social and economic insecurity than in the past.

Despite many legal and social gains over the past 40 years, *inequities persist*. The echoes of inequality in intimate and partnering spaces are tremendously distressing and can be found especially in lopsided statistics on health access and outcomes, home ownership, disability, and intimate partner violence where BIPOC and LGBTQ+ people, and women in general fare worse by many measures.

Those who historically have been on the vulnerable end of the equation in forming any kind of relationship remain there. Unfortunately, kink relationships, like all relationships, exist within this context of persistent inequities.

To put it simply, consent that is compromised feels like:

>> You aren't saying what you mean, need, or want because you're afraid of judgment, shunning, or losing your partner.

>> You are being treated like you're "less-than" by your partner — and this is recognizable because your body and your psyche react.

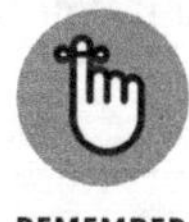

REMEMBER

Consent feels like care. You can feel it in the following ways:

>> You feel great about offering another person your sacred trust. Your partner isn't just trying to get over on or take something from you.

>> Your kink partners give a damn about what you say and none of your needs or feelings are dismissed as problematic or immature.

>> You don't risk your health, your friendships, or your job for this kink. You're not in a situation where your partner(s) fail to address or even notice your vulnerabilities.

The idea of consent among equals doesn't mean that you and your kink partners are all the same. Your lovers don't have to be the same age or race, have the same level of education, possess the same physical or mental abilities, or be living with identical income or resources for you to be playing or partnering with them as an equal. Balancing power as equals means that whatever differences that exist in that mix of realities — you're able to represent yourself and your needs *on par with your play partners.* That none of the differences in these arenas where power often plays out irresponsibly or harmfully have rendered you silent or less worthy or less influential in any discussion of how you create your kink scenarios or take care of your lives.

Creating transparency and accountability

Being truthful and taking full responsibility for your actions (otherwise known as *accountability*, see Appendix A) are core values in kinky communities. *Transparency*, or full disclosure, means that each person is informed about all of the possible issues at play — other relevant relationships in the scenario, physical and mental health issues, as well as your specific kink vulnerabilities and desires.

A simple way to evaluate whether your kink interaction is achieving transparency is this: No one shares or withholds information that would betray trust or harm the other person in the mix.

You know you're in a bad kink situation when something as simple as transparency or honesty becomes unclear or hard to define. No matter how complex your kink desires are, honesty is simple.

PRACTICING FULL DISCLOSURE IN KINK LIFE

Practicing full disclosure involves a certain level of self-awareness. First, you have to know yourself well enough to know when you're lying — perhaps for self-protection or possibly to manipulate others to get what you want. And secondly, you must commit to telling your partner(s) what you know, when you know it. The next exercise explores this concept.

Use your current or a past relationship to consider the following:

>> Do I refuse to look at relationship difficulties and wish them away?

>> Do I hide my emotions and experiences and create confusion?

>> Do I create hidden intimacies with others as a way to escape relationship difficulties?

>> Do I deny what's really going on with me when asked directly?

» Do I pretend not to know things to hide out or deflect responsibility?

» Do I decide major relationship issues without consulting my partner, and then just report on or impose my conclusions?

» Am I the last person to apologize in any given conflict?

If you answered yes to two or more of these questions, you're not in a good place to be accountable and offer full transparency to your kink partners. You likely need more support to heal from wounds that have made you hide yourself and deflect responsibility for your actions. In Chapter 7, you can get more help to grow your capacity to show up and be honest in intimate and kink spaces.

ENCOUNTERING LIES IN KINK RELATIONSHIPS

Being with a partner who lies or deflects responsibility for their actions is painful and dangerous in any relationship. But in kink situations, this type of deception can be even more serious. When you choose to give up or assume power in a kink scenario, if a partner lies about their emotional state or their actions or fails to adhere to your agreements, the result could be serious physical or psychological harm.

WHEN I KNOW, YOU KNOW

One of our favorite kink relational practices is: when I know, you know. When people are struggling in their relationships, they tend to mystify basic truths. A partner will say that they're confused or that something is complex, when the truth is they aren't ready to say the hard thing that they already know. They're afraid of the consequences of their truth — whether a crush on a coworker or how their sexual needs aren't getting met. A common path from this kind of dodge is for a distressed or frightened partner to make a series of bad decisions on their own and then come to their partner with their often-disastrous results — a breach of trust, an affair, or a series of lies.

Relationship coach Asha Leong, one of the many contributors whose stories you'll read in this book, notes that this relationship practice is her most cherished. Everyone struggles to figure themselves out. But holding back what you know because you don't want to deal with a partner's feelings or are worried their response won't align with what you want, isn't honest. In the end, it doesn't protect or help anyone and only reveals a kind of selfishness or disregard that is very hard to recover from. Therefore, a best practice in kink life is: *When I know, you know.*

Of course, no one is perfect. The point is not to be perfect, but to be self-aware. You may stumble in your attempts to inform your partners about your needs in a kink interaction because you have been shamed about this particular desire. You may make mistakes about when to use your safewords or pretend that you are comfortable when you are not.

TIP

The point is to engage as much as possible around tender or gray areas, so you can take the best care of yourself and your play partners or lovers.

WARNING

If lying is habitual for you, or if despite trying to show up honestly, you consistently fail, help is available (see Appendix B). Being dishonest while engaging in kink scenes and building kink relationships is dangerous for you and for your partners.

LYING AT WORK MIGHT MEAN HE'S A DANGEROUS DOM

I had an incredible Dominant (Dom) partner in my 30s whose sexy, authoritarian ways were opening up new worlds for me every time we played. Our intimacy was growing, and I felt safe within the bubble of our kink scenes to take more and more risks. We didn't live together, but our work lives overlapped quite a bit; we often found ourselves on the same community coalition project or campaign.

Over time, I noticed that he did not come through on his commitments as a collaborator. He would say one thing and do another. He deflected responsibility around failing to keep deadlines or complete work we were responsible for collectively. At one meeting, he outright lied about his failure to show up at an event we were all responsible for.

Even though these lies didn't occur in a sexual situation, my playmate's failure to be accountable to the group in this work context eroded my trust in him. I had to stop playing with him. And it was *hard*. I loved our world of kinky play!

But when someone lies consistently — whether about work, money, or picking up the groceries — it's likely that they will eventually fail at keeping their commitments in the sometimes volatile, often demanding theater of kink play. **—Jaime**

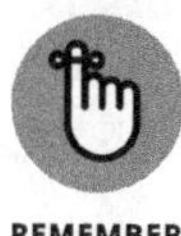

Euphoric states are extremely compelling. Stay awake and keep your eyes open. You are responsible for taking care of you in your kinky life.

A habitual liar is a danger to you.

Exploring mutual respect

An important part of the mutual respect standard among kinksters is that each person's life and well-being in kink play has equal value, even if the relationship is casual or fleeting. *Everyone in a scene is respected* regardless of each player's roles, significance, or meaning in the lives of other players.

Mutual respect in kink play has a kind of breathtaking simplicity, which means

>> You can speak your mind.

>> You're not worrying, rehearsing, or burying important conversations about how you're feeling or what you want.

>> Your limits are respected; your safety needs are met; and your wants are of interest to everyone in the kink interaction.

>> You feel amazing.

While the detailed development of scenes and co-creation of agreements is championed in kink culture, discussion about the elements of mutual respect is a little less prevalent. A way to assess whether mutual respect is upheld in your kink scenes or relationships is to ask yourself:

>> Am I able to be myself here?

>> While there's great talk about equality or respect, do my opinions matter at the same level as my scene partner or lover(s)?

>> Is it really okay to use my safeword, or am I subtly or not so subtly encouraged to meet the needs of one or more others in the scene?

>> Am I afraid of looking uncool or being ousted from a social circle or left alone? Am I afraid to be myself?

Knowing When Consent Is Impossible

When power is not balanced, or the basic humanity of any player is disregarded, or when a kinkster is drunk and not in control of themselves — offering or obtaining consent is not possible. Here is a list of common scenarios where consent isn't even in the realm of possibility:

>> You are my professor or teacher, grading my work.

>> You are my boss or supervisor, filling out my evaluations or signing my paycheck.

>> You are my landlord or caregiver, and I'm relying on you for my home or shelter.

>> You have intimidated or hit me at any time in our relationship.

>> You have isolated me from friends and family and I'm afraid to challenge you.

>> I have ingested substances and I'm not grounded or in a position to make decisions for myself.

In any of these scenarios, regardless of the agreements in effect, consent is compromised by the overwhelming power of one person, or the debilitated condition of another.

These consent fundamentals are your grounding for co-creating great scenes with your lovers and play partners. To build great practices and safely explore your treasured kink fantasies, look to Chapters 4 and 8 for more ideas, kink stories, and guidance.

Chapter 4

Encountering Kinky Worlds

There are countless ways to express your kinky self, an ever-expanding universe of possibility. Kinks that are well-known in the mainstream are just the tip of the kinky iceberg. This chapter presents common kinks so that you can start to identify your interests and consider how you might want to play. But don't think of this as a definitive or complete list. Look to the information here to notice where your passions lie, and then use the activities and inventories in Chapter 5 to build your kinky identity and choose your path.

Perhaps the most widely known kink acronym is *BDSM*, which stands for three revered kink pairings: Bondage and Domination (B & D), Domination and submission (D/s), and Sadism and Masochism (S/M). So, let's start there.

Trying on Bondage and Discipline

Bondage and Discipline (B & D) make up the first two letters of the well-known BDSM moniker as shown in Figure 4-1.

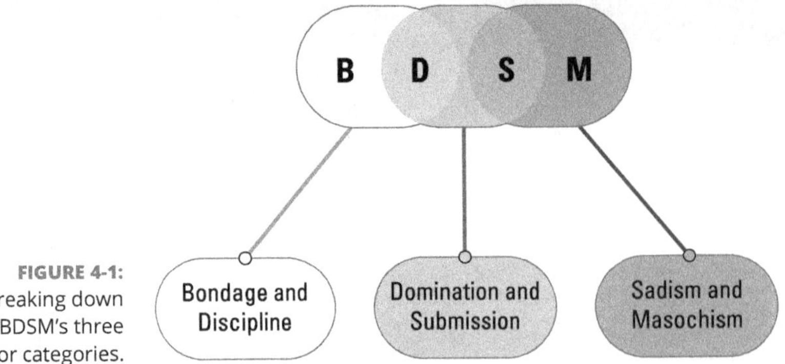

FIGURE 4-1: Breaking down BDSM's three major categories.

This section provides foundational information on bondage and discipline as a core category of kink desire: What is it? What do people experience when playing with Bondage and Discipline?

Bondage basics

Whether a rope bunny or a tape mummifier, bondage aficionados report the same: it's incredibly gratifying to restrain or be restrained by their playmates. *Rope Masters* (highly skilled rope bondage practitioners) may be entranced by the intricacies and beauty of their work; sometimes they are as enthralled by their dedication to learning the complexities of the knots as the effect that the work has on their partners. A mummification *submissive* (also known as a sub or bottom) may be aroused by the high level of trust they invest in their *Dominant* (a Dom or Top; see the section, "Exploring Domination and Submission" later in this chapter) and their experience of total surrender. Gratification can be multilayered, just like the practices themselves.

Holding someone down or tying them up

Bondage doesn't have to be complex. Depending on your partner, holding a lover down by their wrists or simply tying back their arms with a canvas belt can create just as much excitement as an elaborate scene in kink play. (Silk scarves can tighten and be hard to unknot — so despite what your favorite erotica says, don't use them).

TIP

The simple certainty of restraint — like being *encaged* (perhaps against a wall or in missionary position in bed) in a partner's arms — and the surrender it requires may be all that is needed to engage a partner's bondage kink.

Even so, bondage has so many interesting and elaborate forms including:

>> **Cuffs:** Handcuffed to the bedframe is a classic, observed in so many great porn and mainstream movies. Despite the ubiquitousness of metal cuffs in the movies, most kinksters prefer a padded cuff to increase comfort and longevity of a scene (see Figure 4-2).

>> **Spreader bars:** Spreader bars are another immobilizing option that many love for the increased vulnerability that the bar creates, by requiring you to spread your arms or legs, for cuffing to a bar.

>> **Rope play:** In rope bondage (shown in Figure 4-3), some kinksters find the binding itself to be the main event for gratification. Others employ the various ties as a restrictive prelude to genital sex, where the immobilization of the roped kinkster creates heightened arousal and easy access.

In terms of material, braided cotton or nylon are preferred for their price point, comfort, and ease of undoing. They can also be cheaply accessed at a local hardware store. Thinner ropes can hurt and are more likely to harm nerve endings.

>> **Shibari:** As a highly favored Japanese rope binding practice, shibari uses single and double column ties to provide a gateway into a complex and compelling aesthetic world of ties. Hemp and jute are preferred materials for shibari, pricier than cotton or nylon but more comfortable and durable with minimal stretch.

>> **Nautical or seafaring ties:** Associated with sailing and boating, these ties are popular, and training is easily accessed via in-person classes or online.

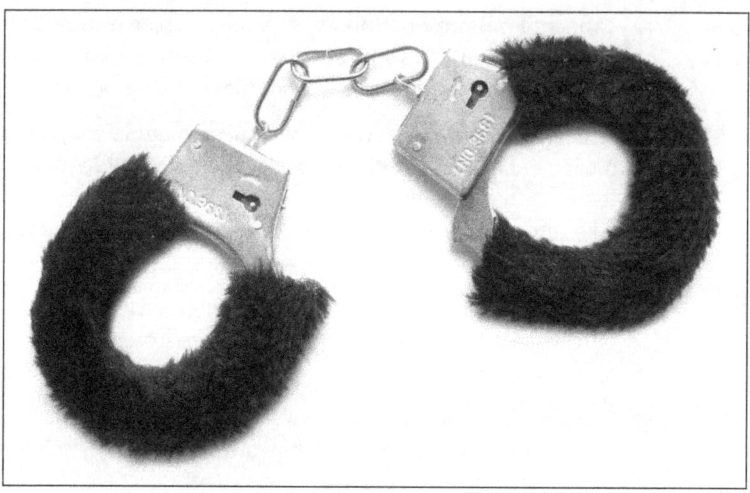

FIGURE 4-2:
Fuzzy handcuffs.

© *Yulliash/Adobe Stock photos*

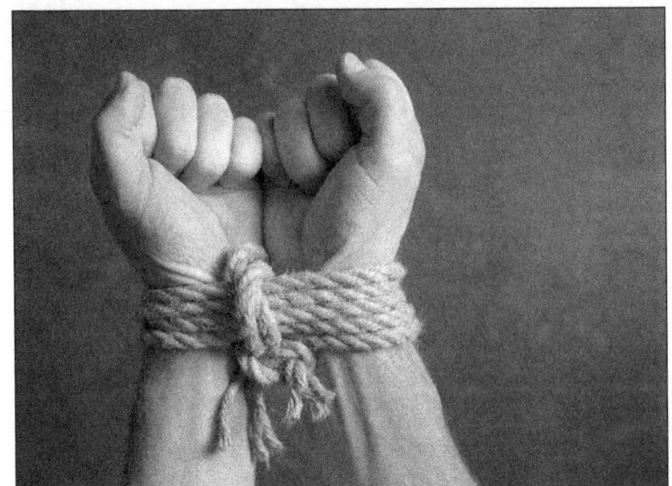

FIGURE 4-3:
Simple wrist tie.

>> **Suspension rope work:** Rigging, or suspending a play partner who is immobilized in knots, is a form of play that requires significant training. Hemp and jute are preferred for suspension rope work; minimal stretch and the stability of the knots are important to safety.

If you fantasize about binding or being bound, a huge community of enthusiasts and practitioners awaits you.

WARNING

As a rope Top, always have serrated medical shears with you at all times, not just a knife. And never leave someone who is in any kind of bondage alone.

>> **Tape and mummification:** Wrist or ankle taping provide quick-and-easy bondage for kinksters who are after quick restraint without a lot of ritual and is often great for calling up fantasies of being captured.

Mummification involves wrapping a sub in material that restricts their movement altogether; it's usually head to toe with breathing holes or neck to toe so that the sub's head is unrestricted. Mummifying with bondage tape takes time and skill. For kinksters who love the ritual of bondage, mummification with tape, rope, and plastic wrap is prized.

WARNING

Old school duct tape is not safe for bondage. Instead, you will want to purchase bondage tape from a sex or crafts store, at least 2 inches wide and made of PVC.

>> **Sleep sacks or body bags:** Sleep sacks are totally and instantly immobilizing. If you want to minimize the time involved in highly restrictive bondage while maximizing the constraint effect, body bags may be for you. These sacks zip you into a compressed space, with collars that buckle around the neck, and internal sleeves for the arms. While in the sack, you have no access to any part of your body. (Jack offers his experience of body bags in Chapter 2.)

Sensory deprivation: masks and hoods

Some kinksters like to lose visual, auditory, or other forms of contact with the world around them during a scene. Simple masks, a tied scarf blindfold (see Figure 4-4), leather hoods, ear plugs — any of these can inhibit or eliminate one of your senses so that you can be more present with yourself or more dependent on your scene partner.

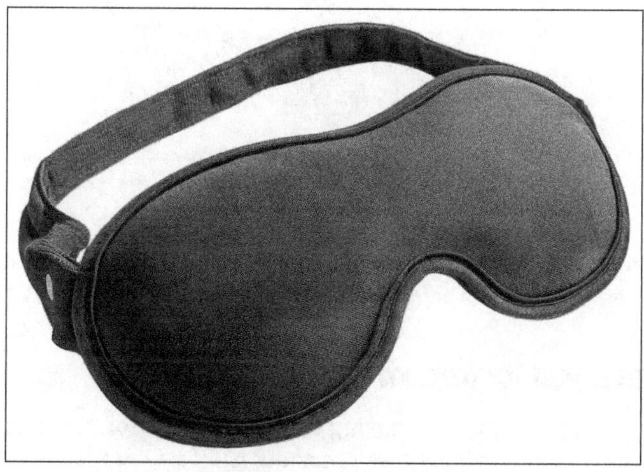

FIGURE 4-4: Basic mask.

© Saim Art/Adobe Stock Photos

One kink player noted: *I enjoy sensory deprivation, and the limitation of my connection to the outside world. I can turn inward and pay attention to myself for a change. And losing access to my phone is just as profound as not being able to see or hear.*

Ball and bit gags

Similar to sensory deprivation, some kinksters like to restrict the way they can express themselves while in a scene. Different kinds of gags will partially or totally inhibit speech. Additionally, a gag can move a submissive into a desired state of pleasurable discomfort.

Gags come in variety of styles and shapes. A ball gag (as shown in Figure 4-5) involves a silicone or rubber ball strapped to the head and held in the mouth. Another common form is the rolled chord bit gag, reminiscent of the metal bits used in horses' mouths. Gags also come in shapes that force the mouth open or otherwise create access for a Dom to insert objects or body parts while restricting speech and facial movement.

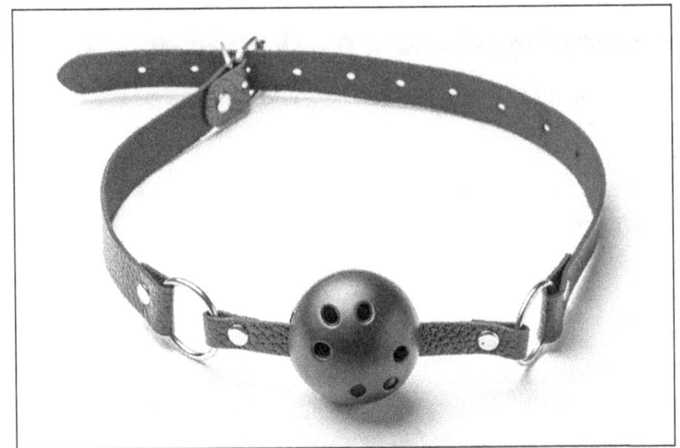

FIGURE 4-5:
Classic ball gag.

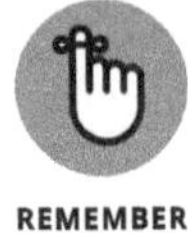

REMEMBER

Remember to choose a simple nonverbal safeword or safe action if you're playing with someone who is gagged and can't speak (see Chapter 8).

Cages and locked rooms

Kinksters may appreciate having reduced options for movement, such as a cage, including for puppy play (see Appendix A). If you are looking for simplicity, just being locked in a closet may do the trick. Similar to other forms of bondage, kinksters report relief and gratification at having their mobility severely restricted. An example of a cage is shown in Figure 4-6.

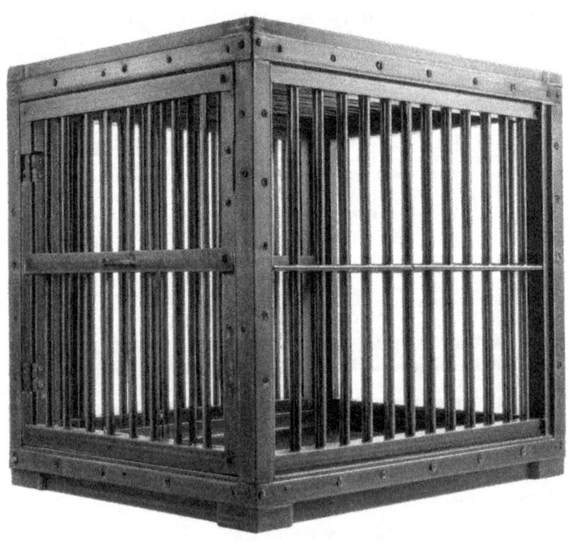

FIGURE 4-6:
Confinement
cage.

Cock cages, chastity belts, and genital control

Restraint of the genitals is a highly prized kind of bondage, and often involves orgasm control (see Appendix A). Locking up the penis in a cock cage or barring access to the vagina and clitoris via a chastity belt can create a sense of ownership between partners and give the Dom complete control over their partner's pleasure, including access to self-pleasure.

If you are like us, and you lose things a lot, especially your keys — having a second key that you store in a fixed location is a great way to take care of you and your partners.

Enacting discipline

Disciplinary kink calls up imaginary, historic, and actual terrors around various kinds of punishments children and people who survive captivity have endured. For example, caning as a kink disciplinary practice emerged from corporal punishment experienced by children in various public and private schools over millennia and has been thus inscribed in the kink imagination.

Inside the B & D scene, discipline involves rule-making and sometimes behavior modification followed by praise or punishment. Correction occurs when clear expectations have been outlined and set for a scene or a contract, and the sub defies or fails to meet those expectations. What follows are a number of commonly practiced forms of discipline.

Withdrawing attention and other penalties

Doms may employ a variety of strategies to discipline their playmates, including infantilizing time-outs, withdrawing attention, placing an offending bottom in the corner or a closet, writing judgments on the skin, forcing subs to maintain punishing poses, and so on.

Classic reprimands stimulate humiliation, grief, and self-reproach in the submissive, releasing that sought-after surge in the release of endorphins, a morphine-like chemical in the brain that triggers pleasure and pain relief.

Spanking

Spanking is a highly popular form of disciplinary or impact play. It can be enacted on a sub who is fully clothed, in underwear, or naked. The recipient can be positioned over the knee or standing or laid out. Over the knee is a treasured classic in kink play.

It's best to be able to continuously check the impact of the spanking if you are going to do an extended spanking scene. Clothing can often extend the course of play because it reduces sting and direct impact, while also impairing your ability to monitor impact.

While many prefer to use a hand to spank a partner, paddlers and slappers are also commonly used. These come in all shapes and sizes, with leather, wood, silicone among favored materials. Paddlers and slappers can be multilayered and customized with your scene names or a favorite degrading label. A paddle (see Figure 4-7) may be preferred by the Dom or sub in question for the particular patterning it leaves on the receiver.

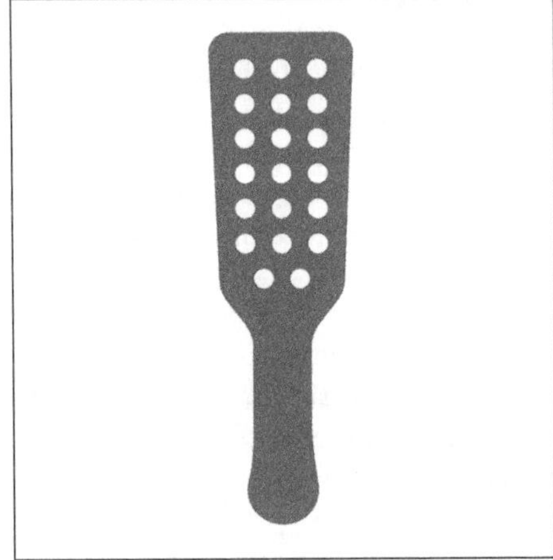

FIGURE 4-7:
Classic paddle.

© amin268/Adobe Stock Photos

Whipping and caning are also often used as disciplinary measures, and you can find them described in the "Investigating Sadism and Masochism" section later in this chapter.

Spanking best practice: move your hand over the impacted area after hitting, to assess impact, soothe, and increase pleasure for both parties.

Noticing how much control you need

Like all kink practices, B & D is an exercise in finding the range of action or intersections where you and your scene partner's desires meet. For example, your ideal restraint scenario may be at a more complex or constraining level than that of the partner you are excited about tying up. Your high need for punishment may be beyond the capacity or tolerance of your Dom. One of the great joys of kinky play is the process of meeting each person where they are and figuring out how to create a satisfying dynamic.

You may need to try a lot of different scenes with a partner to find a sweet spot that satisfies both of your desires for control and surrender.

The joy of letting go

Kinksters who long to be on the receiving end of B & D are often (but not always) people who are shouldering enormous responsibility in their daily lives. They describe their experiences of being immobilized (see Figure 4-8) or punished as enormously relieving or joyful.

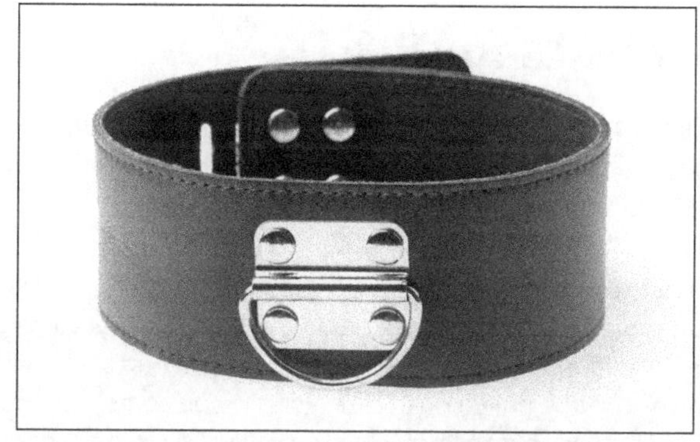

FIGURE 4-8:
Cuffs to
immobilize.

© Tiler84/Adobe Stock Photos

Many report trance-like states of ecstasy. This is often referred to as *subspace* — a submissive state of letting go where one is literally floating on a sea of hormonal bliss induced by the inability to move, act, or do (see Chapter 9).

Alternatively, some B & D lovers are already in situations of powerlessness all day long; they have terrible bosses or may be trapped in an abusive marriage. In these cases, playing out punishing or helpless scenarios can be liberating precisely because they *are play* and not reality. You can meticulously create the terms of your B & D scenes, the starting and stopping points, which is the opposite of your real-life experience.

Playing with and upending gender norms is a powerful form of kink play with a long history around the world. Men and other masculine-identified subs report getting a particular charge from worshipping women or submitting to their will in ways that goes against the scripts they've been required to follow in public life. This is such a popular kink that many women make a living as professional Dominatrixes (See Appendix A).

Examples of the way masculine subs play this out include kissing feet, heels, or hosiery; worshipping genitals; being verbally demeaned about their masculinity, penis, or sexual performance; and submitting to pain dictated by the whims of a woman or femme. They may also agree to be "sissified" or feminized by their Tops as a path to pleasurable humiliation.

Safety basics for B & D

While Chapters 3 and 8 provide great grounding in building consent and complex kinky scenes that safely pursue your wants, there are a few specifics to note for safety when exploring Bondage and Discipline.

>> **Pay attention to your body.** If you've done a good job co-creating the terms of your scene, you and your partner know what physical vulnerabilities require attention in your play together. Have you had shoulder surgery so your arms can't be pulled on in restraint? Do you sometimes have panic attacks and need to stop to reset your nervous system or your breathing? Pay attention.

>> **Make sure your safewords are accessible.** Some bondage — like masks or ball gags, or in some cases being tied up or taped — can inhibit verbal communication, so be sure to create alternative safety protocols in these situations. If your hands are free, tapping your scene partner or waving can work. Remember that your safeword substitute, your *all-stop action,* must be simple and instantly recognizable to your partner.

>> **Materials matter.** Trial and error with the materials of Bondage and Discipline can be important. You want the marks left by a rope bondage or a whip to linger in a pleasurable way, not hurtful or damaging.

>> **Don't overextend yourself.** Attending to your limits can be a tricky thing to navigate when you are swept up in the joy of either restraining or surrender-ing to your partner. Their delight can persuade you to abandon yourself. You wouldn't want your partner to ignore their emotional or physical vulnerabili-ties, causing harm to themselves. So take care of yourself just as seriously.

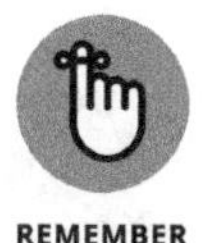

You aren't a better or cooler B & D enthusiast by ignoring your limits in service to your partner's pleasure.

Exploring Domination and Submission

Domination and submission make up the middle two letters of the fabled BDSM acronym, usually written as D/s as shown in Figure 4-1 at the beginning of the chapter.

In this section, you can explore how people who have a desire to control or dominate their partners work to make these fantasies a reality. At the same time, you can discover various ways people choose to give up control or submit to an authoritative scene partner to satisfy their kinky longings.

Taking or surrendering power

The core dynamic in D/s play is that one person controls or directs the scene and the other surrenders control or submits. The D/s dynamic is so ubiquitous in movies and literature that you can literally find it anywhere, from bodice-ripping romance novels to hardcore porn. When you think about it, D/s is more or less the foundation for "normative" gender roles within a conservative gender order or society.

D/s kinksters want to dig deeply into the Domination and submission dynamic. They want to push the envelope far past what we see in rom-coms.

Below, are a number of common ways that kinksters play out their D/s yearnings.

Bratting, humiliation, and praise kinks

D/s kinksters may play out a range of emotive and temperamental dynamics. Here are a few:

>> **Bratting.** A favorite in D/s play space involves what we think of as attitudinal play. Some subs love to be bratty with their Doms. Brat behavior elicits a hot, corrective response from them.

For subs who have a particularly hard time surrendering their power, bratting — and the actions it evokes — can be a helpful vehicle for flipping that switch and surrendering.

>> **Humiliation play.** Also a hugely popular D/s avenue, kinksters may create humiliation scenes that have been discussed at length. They might describe the origins of that need (if they know it) so that the Dom might push on a particularly vulnerable emotional button that the sub has described.

Small penis humiliation is an example of this (SPH; see Appendix A), wherein a kinkster has been shamed about or is ambivalent about their penis size and confides in a Dom partner who can push on that in a scene, activating and releasing this shame for their sub.

>> **Praise kinks.** This type of play gets a little less attention in the world of attitudinal play, and are explored expansively in fan fiction and pet play. Subs with praise kinks go fuzzy at the litany of "good boy" or "good girl" that fall from the lips of a Dom who is petting them while on a leash. Others might enact office worker scenes where the boss exclaims over their excellent spreadsheets. For many kinksters who have grown up or currently live in a world with little praise, eliciting unending praise from a hot, caring Dom can be wildly gratifying.

Service

Service (or service bottoming) is a widely practiced kink wherein a sub is pleased or aroused by cleaning your apartment, or carrying your bag, or setting up an auditorium for a speech you are about to give. Service can be focused on small daily acts of care or highly choreographed events. For the Top, directing and setting the terms of service, and receiving this care can be extremely satisfying.

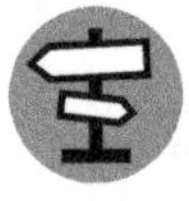

One cute story is that on my birthday, my service sub got me a very nice pair of boots, leather boots that I picked out. And then, at the end of my very demanding semester, he got us an Airbnb — a lovely house in the woods for a week — and he drove my various partners back and forth. He also did all the shopping and just sort of took care of everything. So that was really awesome for me as his Dom, and really satisfying for him. —**Anonymous**

Breath play

Breath play involves controlling the breath of a partner or giving up the control of your breathing.

If this sounds dangerous, that's because it certainly is.

While choking has become kind of ubiquitous on the Internet, and young people talk about it casually like it's entry-level sex play, kinksters who love breath play know differently.

Learning how to appropriately inhibit breath is crucial; I don't recommend this to kink beginners or even experienced kinksters if you are with partners you don't know well.

Safe breath play means you have a partner who is an accomplished kinkster with significant training, including CPR and First Aid, and also is a great communicator who knows your body. Together you have:

>> An excellent consent container and a physical cue to stop all play. A common way to do this is to have your partner hold your hand while they restrict your breathing, and pulling your hand away is your all-stop action.

>> A strong history of trust and success with boundaries together.

>> A kinkster who can describe the anatomy of breath play and what kind of damage they can do if they are not careful.

Final caveat: autoerotic asphyxiation, or doing breath play solo, often to stimulate orgasm, is a significant kink. If this is your fantasy, I can't say be careful strongly enough. Finding others who love this kink, and who can discuss how they create fail-safes, or all stops for themselves is crucial. People die of autoerotic asphyxiation every year. If you don't want others to know about your kink, seek help with safety via anonymous online community.

Daddy or Mommy play

Playing with the Daddy role in kink play has got to be in the top 10 of all time kinks, across every demographic you can name. Mommy play is much less common, but no less powerful for its devotees.

The power of playing with the ultimate incest taboo creates an unparalleled experience for many kinksters.

Non-kinksters can get very get icked-out about this taboo because, as is common, they are thinking about this in literal terms. But playing in this realm isn't about fantasizing about your actual parents. Instead, it's about entering the realm of powerlessness that children experience.

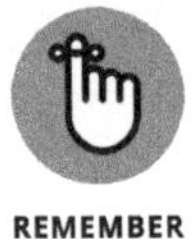

There are few people in life that have total control over you like a parent. Kinksters find joy and release by turning themselves over to this kind of control in Mommy and Daddy play. Mommies and Daddies experience tremendous gratification in being entrusted with the ultimate care of their little ones.

And, as a counterpoint to childhood, you get to choose the temperament of your Mommy or Daddy as a Dom or sub. This can be wonderfully corrective or an intense replay, depending on your kinky needs.

Devastation play and consensual non-consent

Devastation play and consensual non-consent are practices that draw on scenarios that are deeply harmful in real life, and this draws criticism from outsiders because on a basic human level, it feels wrong.

The short sightedness of these well-meaning critiques is that they assess kink play logically, and they fail to account for our unconscious life, which absorbs a plethora of painful events and performs a kind of *alchemy of desire* (when you throw all of your harms and yearnings into the fire of lust and connection, something new and unexpected gets made.)

In this place of transformation, your experiences of harm can imprint on your sexuality and desire and re-emerge as deep longings and a yearning to connect. Nowhere are these complexities more contested than in devastation play such as Master/slave scenarios, and consensual non-consent or rape play, which we'll discuss below.

Playing Master/slave

There's only one redeeming truth about the history of slavery in the U.S. and around the world, and that is the history of resistance by enslaved people, and their unrelenting efforts to survive and protect themselves and their families.

This is the territory that is mined in Master/slave (M/s) scenarios among kinksters whose families have either survived enslavement or enslaved people. Given the lasting impact and overlay of slavery in the U.S. culture, Master/slave play is tremendously powerful for both descendants of enslaved people and enslavers, as well as those whose family story lives outside of that history. Accordingly, some kinksters find it to be their most explosive, and thus treasured, place of play. Others find it absolutely distasteful and out of the realm of possibility.

In a Master/slave play dynamic, the "slave" gives over total power to the Dom in this master role. Through M/s play, subs experience a euphoria in offering absolute control to the Dom for the duration of the scene, and the "Master" experiences a parallel gratification for being entrusted so completely with their sub's well-being. Strong consent container creation is paramount in M/s play (see Chapters 3 and 8).

Master/slave kinksters report loving the unqualified surrender in this play arena and the intensity of the taboo. Subs may enjoy being in charge of the co-creation of the scenes, which is a reversal of actual M/s relationships in history where the enslaved held no power to dictate the terms of their daily lives.

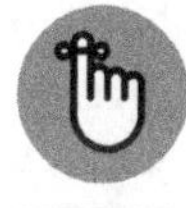

REMEMBER

If Master/slave play is compelling and healthy for you and your partners, your scenes and your daily life will feel full and freeing. If Master/slave play is harmful to you, the opposite will occur. Your history and/or the emotional demands of the power exchange will be damaging, and you will need to stop, and reassess.

Sometimes, this play is healthy for a kinkster for a period, and then it becomes toxic or depleting without any kind of warning or specific problem in a scene. The same caveat holds for consensual non-consent play, described below.

TIP

Pay close attention to your condition, even if you've been engaging in M/s play over time.

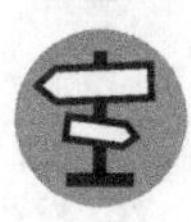

KINK STORY

I'm a Black, queer, trans feminist . . . and I enjoy playing Master in M/s play. On the surface, that might seem like a contradiction — how can someone committed to justice desire something so loaded, so historically violent? But my kink life isn't about replicating that history. It's about reclaiming power and flipping the narrative.

My wanting a slave isn't about superiority. A slave isn't someone lesser — they're someone willing to meet me in raw, devoted intimacy. That intimacy demands just as much from me as it does from them. The responsibility is real. The care is real. And that complexity — the tension between what I resist in the world and what I embrace in the dungeon — isn't a contradiction to me. It's not about domination rooted in harm. It's about power rooted in care. **—Shaan**

Building consensual non-consent

Consensual non-consent (CNC) means that the parties involved choreograph a scene where one person forces sex upon the other without discussion or warning, but in a manner that has been *previously agreed to and meticulously outlined together.* CNC play is controversial at a comparable level to M/s play and just as strongly held by kinksters who treasure it.

Many people who play with rape in their kink scenes are survivors of sexual assault, and many are not. Again, this kind of play appears to be an unhealthy avenue of play for a survivor of violence, but only if one believes that CNC scenes are impossible to construct collaboratively.

In effect, consensual non-consent scenes upend the terms of sexual violence and abuse by putting all of the choices in the hands of the sub or bottom.

Like M/s play, kinksters who are passionate about this play — whether they are survivors or not — report cathartic relief and immense gratification from this scripted, highly charged, intimate power-exchange.

One of the most powerful tools in my healing was consensual non-consent. I needed to shift the power that nonconsensual harm still held over me. So, I eroticized it — on my own terms. In scenes crafted with deep care and trust, I allowed my body to reenact what once overwhelmed me. Only this time, I chose it. I orchestrated it. I ended it when I needed.

The terror was still there — but so was the arousal, the control, the reclamation. It was hot. It was healing. In that space, I wasn't a victim — *I was a force.* CNC let me flirt with my fear, hold it in my mouth, moan through it, and still walk away whole. That is what devastation play gave me: not pain, but power. **—Ignacio**

Navigating devastation and CNC kinks

Newcomers to kink often ask: what's the difference between a healthy and an unhealthy kink? When is a passion or desire for a certain kind of play over the line or too much? This often seems like a complicated question because the scenes you may be lusting after are complex or wade into devastating historic or emotional territories like enslavement or rape.

But the test for whether or not any kink is working for you is startlingly simple. Take the following basic inventory:

> » Are you happy?

> » Is your kink play bringing wonderful, trustworthy people into your life?

> » Do you feel lighter, joyful, or lucky?

Or

>> Is life heavier?

>> Do you feel confused or conflicted?

>> Do you find yourself unable to contain the impacts of a CNC or a Master/slave scene? Are your aftercare practices failing to bring you back to a functioning level in daily life?

>> Is your self-esteem suffering?

>> Is your work or family life suffering?

>> Are you putting your job or your partnership in jeopardy because of your attachment to this kind of play?

If you said no to one or two of the top three questions and yes to more than one of the bottom six, then devastation play is not working for you.

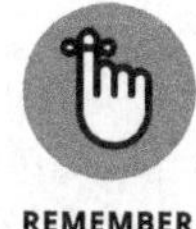

This assessment doesn't mean this kind of play can never work for you, but you need to be honest with yourself that it's not working for you now.

Mitigating potential for harm

If you find that devastation or consensual non-consent play is actually harming you or causing you to physically or emotionally dissemble, it's time to stop, reassess, and take care of yourself. Sometimes it means:

>> Putting CNC back in the fantasy column for a while, or even forever.

>> Having more discussion among kinksters who also play in M/s and CNC territories to learn how they handle their emotional lives in the aftermath.

>> Noting a particular reaction you had that disrupted the scene to assess what this means to you. Perhaps you need to focus on more healing or maybe you and your Dom need to improve your communication skills.

>> Understanding that sometimes intense scenes go perfectly well in the moment, and then you "drop" or experience an intense emotional impact hours or days later (see Chapter 9).

While this applies to any arena of play, keeping an eye out for harm is particularly important in CNC and M/s play, where the emotional and physical stakes are high.

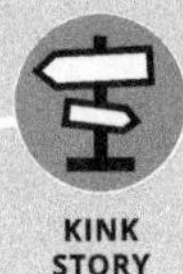

YOU'RE OPEN RIGHT?

When I moved to Indiana for grad school, I met a tall, country white dude with blonde hair, blue eyes and bulky beard on a well-known app and whenever we'd discuss our various kinks, he'd repeatedly ask "You're open, right?" I assured him I was. I invited him over and while we were starting to get busy, he stopped, went over to his bookbag and began pulling out what looked like a white sheet which confused me. Again, he prompted "You said you're open right?" to which I nodded with a mix of curiosity and confusion. At that point, I noticed that the sheet had three distinct holes but before I could process what was happening, he smirked and confidently revealed, "Well, I'm into race play, and I want to fuck you like the n***** you are."

I found the strength to go to the kitchen of my studio apartment and grab the largest knife I could find before loudly responding, "Oh you're into race play, huh? Well, let's role-play the Haitian Revolution then!" He cursed at me, grabbed his clothes and ran out the door.

After meeting a second guy who also moved into race play without any negotiation, I became completely emotionally detached and shut down altogether, for two years. Looking back, subconsciously I knew that any attempt to deal with the weight of my feelings would likely prevent me from finishing graduate school. **—Kamilah**

SEXUAL SHOPLIFTING

D/s play doesn't happen on neutral territory. So many actual, destructive power plays are unfolding daily in our lives. As I've noted in other chapters, a lot of kinksters play in these problematic arenas in an attempt to reverse or transform harm that has happened to them.

A *sexual shoplifter* is someone who fails to account for these imbalances in their play, risking nothing while facilitating actual harm. For example:

- A man who uses degrading language with women or femme playmates and works in an organization that blocks women's access to employment or health care.

- A straight partner who enjoys doing hate crime scenes with gay men and votes for anti-gay laws.

Predator/prey

The Predator/prey play dynamic hinges on the Dom holding psychological power or a specific reward, and the sub feeling small or vulnerable and being required to navigate concrete risks to please the Dom or to be rewarded. Many kinksters love playing out Predator/prey online or by text, and others enjoy developing complicated in-person scenarios. A mix of these is described here.

>> **Spider/fly interactions:** Spider/fly interactions are all about the headgame. Heeeerrreee, kitty, kitty. Come to your Dom. I have some lovely fresh milk here for you, and if you take it, I'll reward you with your favorite way to be gratified, but I might also lock you in this kitty cage and leave you. Spider/fly interactions generally involve a reward that the Dom is enticingly holding out, and a risk that the sub must navigate to get it.

>> **Surveillance:** Jaime once had a Dom who asked her to share her location on her phone with him. She had never considered this in kink play and asked him what happened to him when he got a phone notification of her movements. He replied that he got instantly aroused. She asked "like, every time?" He said yes. As a sub, this gave Jaime an enormous sense of power and exhilaration as she moved through her day; she was turning on her Dom just by traveling across town to a meeting. It also left her feeling vulnerable. Would her Dom show up somewhere unannounced? Did he judge where she ate for lunch as bad and would he enact a punishment? Surveillance play with a trustworthy Dom can be incredibly hot.

>> **Kidnapping:** Kidnapping scenarios are complex. Obviously, doing them in public can draw attention and get you into serious trouble. So, *safety first!* Many kinksters love creating very detailed consent and scene containers (see Chapters 3 and 8) for kidnapping scenes, and then leave the actual timing up to the Dom so that the sub is truly surprised. In this kind of scenario, both parties can be maximally gratified by the various spontaneous variables that play out. If we were talking about D/s in academic terms, we would say kidnapping requires an advanced degree level of knowing yourself and navigating your kinks — not for the novice.

Group or public sex

Having sex out in the open, in view of or with others is part and parcel of a number of prized kinks within the D/s construct. If you feel drawn to group scenes, playing with self-display or displaying your partners, and flipping emotionally between pride and humiliation, these kinks might be yours.

Voyeurism and exhibitionism

If you find yourself turned on when observing public displays of affection, or generally compelled by visuals in your arousal, *voyeurism* may be one of your kinks. Consensual voyeurism can be enjoyed at kink clubs and play parties, where the guidelines for watching are explicitly stated. The great benefit of clubs and parties is that you get to see many kinds of kink interactions and displays all at once, which can give you a lot of information about what you are into.

On the flip side of the coin, if you've always loved being the center of attention, or conversely, have felt somewhat ashamed or vulnerable being the center of attention, *exhibitionism* might be your jam. A simple way to lean into your exhibitionist tendencies is to try them out with a lover or trusted scene partner. Talking through a simple strip tease or defining a scene where you get naked and clean the apartment for an appreciative audience can be a great starting place.

Outside of kink spaces, trying out voyeurism in cruising parks is trickier around safety but also widely practiced. Taking a wing person or play partner with you to a cruising spot can greatly increase your safety while you are figuring out how things operate in the space.

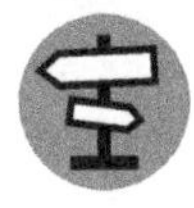

A few years back, I stumbled upon this wild sex party in Washington DC. The energy was *electric* and as I was mingling, I started noticing all these couples and groups getting down and dirty, having fun with flirtation and playful romantic sexual activities, and I was like, *yasssss*.

I felt a spark inside me — a new interest in watching others. I started helping out the party attendants by handing out condoms, water, and all sorts of sex toys. Every time I handed someone a toy or a pack of condoms, I felt this surge of excitement. It was like I was part of the magic, helping bring people together. It was a major thrill to see all these connections being formed around me. I was right in the middle of this beautiful, messy, fantastic atomic bond, and I loved every minute of it. Seeing how happy and curious others are lit a voyeurism fire in me, uncovering a part of myself I didn't even know was there. **—Anonymous**

Clothed person, naked person

Some kinksters enjoy being the only naked person in the pairing, or even the room. This kink involves lusting after your own authority or the vulnerability of the naked person in the kink scenario, or conversely, enjoying the feeling of being exposed or in "jeopardy" relative to the clothed kinkster. Enthusiasts often label this play by gender using terms like CFNM (clothed female, naked male) or CMNM (clothed male, naked male).

Cuckolding, hotwifing, and watching

Cuckolding is the practice of consensually offering your partner to another person for sex and enjoying the sense of humiliation you feel while observing them together. Sometimes this occurs within larger public view, or you may offer your partner to several others in a scene. A newer term, hotwifing, is an offshoot of cuckolding, wherein the "husband" who offers his "wife" feels pride rather than humiliation in this exchange. (We use quotes here because people of any gender and in any relationship form can offer or be offered in this prideful scenario.) In a heterosexual context, hotwifing has also been described as a form of emotional or sexual bonding between men, sometimes referred to as bro bonding.

Free use

When a sub consents to being sexually available at all times to their Dom, without conversation or a reaffirmation of consent in the moment, that agreement is described as free use. Some partners may have exceptions such as *not while we are eating* or *never when the kids are in the house*. Some Doms may secure additional terms of consent to extend the free use "card" to their friends, or partygoers, if that is in keeping with the sub's desires. Free use subs love this kink for the sense of constant anticipation it creates with their Doms; while Dom practitioners describe the joy of being the absolute ruler of their domain, literal king of their "castle" or sub.

Creating your own D/s construct

We could spend a whole book writing about D/s constructs. Do you love a hot cop/escaped convict scene? Or is homeowner/lawn boy more your style? Is it all about the *DILFs* (Dads I Would Love to F*ck)/boys-or-girls-next-door for you? (See Appendix A for help with terms.) Maybe you've never found your specific D/s fantasy anywhere and you need to build your own! Kinksters are endlessly creative.

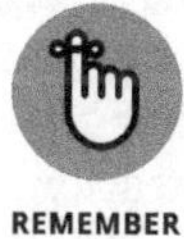

Scripting scenes that correspond to your compelling fixations is a liberating process. If elaborate scenes appeal to you, check out the section "Setting Up Roleplay and Fantasy" later in this chapter. And let your kinky self live!

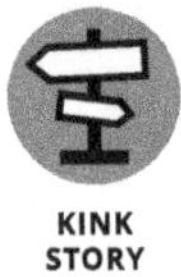

The kind of dominance I get the most charge out of is finding and then "molding" a sub's desire. I had a playmate who knew she was submissive but hadn't explored enough to know which lane of the kink world she was in. I could see that she really liked to please me, so I introduced her to the idea of service and pretty soon she was taking over all kinds of bureaucratic tasks in my life and totally getting off on it. And what I was getting off on was having found her correct lane and putting her in it. With another sub, I took it further by pushing him past his "natural" lane. He's also more identified with service but letting me inflict pain upon him is a kind of service I highly value so that's what we do. He isn't turned on by the pain, in fact he dreads it, but he *is* turned on by the dread and very gratified by the idea that by the end of the session, he's taken care of my needs. —**Anonymous**

Safety basics for D/s

Safety basics for D/s play are similar to safety basics for all play that involves an exchange of power:

>> **For Dominants,** the intoxication or joy experienced when being fully trusted to orchestrate scenes or even the day-to-day events of a sub's life can be overwhelming. It might seem like there can be no downside to this, but it's a lot of responsibility, especially when enacting devastation or nonconsensual consent play. Some Doms have a hard time saying: *This is too much. I can't hold this much power and stay with this scene. Or, I love going there with you, but afterwards, I have a hard time attending to my daily demands at work or in my family. I need to rebalance the terms of our exchange.*

>> **For subs,** the ecstatic state of letting go can lead to a kind of sub gluttony (We are speaking from experience!). You may feel a level of relief you've never felt anywhere else and just want to do more, more, more. It may be wise to try out new levels of submission in gradual doses. Then, you can spend some time after, when you are putting yourself back together and attending to daily life, to assess whether this is a healthy level of relinquishment for you, or if you've verged into a territory that is not sustainable.

Investigating Sadism and Masochism

Like consensual non-consent and various kinds of devastation play (see section earlier in this chapter), sadism and masochism (S/M) is widely read as violent and problematic by the casual observer or non-kinky public. And, like these other intense theaters of kink play, S/M is sought after and appreciated for creating exhilarating, euphoric states of being for its many practitioners and fans.

This section examines the basics of S/M to help you consider whether these compelling kink practices are right for you.

Sadism 101: Sadists come in all flavors

Sadists like inflicting pain. They enjoy watching the impact of their powerful emotional and physical acts on their grateful masochists. They are aroused by the power they hold. They are gripped and transported by the unpredictable effects of any carefully choreographed scene. They love the drama. Above all, they cherish the deep trust their partners extend to them, the connection.

And contrary to popular belief, sadists come in every temperament imaginable, from shy to brash, talkative to silent, brutal to tender. What kind of sadist might you want to be?

Masochism 101: pain is vehicle

In masochistic life, pain is a transportive vehicle, not a harmful dead end. "Pain pigs" clamor after what the pain *generates* for them psychically and physically, not the pain itself. A masochist may find that the rhythmic thudding of a flogger lifts them out of the dreary demands of daily life and throws them into a floating elation that bends time. Or the sting of a single tail whip cracks a veneer of control and complacency that they cannot disrupt by any other means. Or the pain caused by a line of clothes pins attached to their genitals demands full attention, blocking out all other crises and responsibilities.

Varieties of S/M

What the casual observer entirely misses about S/M is its deceptive simplicity: by pursuing or purveying pain, the kinkster in question co-creates an alternative universe that is (literally) awestruck. The chemicals released in the S/M exchange — adrenaline and endorphins — create a euphoric cloud for the participating kinksters. Here are some common SM activities designed to bring about that chaotic, swirling joy.

Impact play

It's the landing that S/M practitioners seek in impact play. How is this activity affecting the body and emotional state of the scene partner? The actions, sounds, visuals, and trust exchange all combine to generate pleasure.

>> **Spanking, whipping and caning:** These three highly prized kink practices all live under both the disciplinary and the sadism umbrellas. Spanking is discussed in the section, "Enacting discipline," earlier in the chapter, so I'll focus on whipping and caning here.

- **Whips and crops:** So many options. Bullwhips or single-tail whips, racing crops, bats and *quirts* (a short riding whip) can all be employed to intense effect. Bullwhips and single tail hits are outrageously impactful, and the endorphin release instantaneous. Whips are not for beginners, Train, train, train. Practice, practice.

  Crops and quirts are quite stingy. If you want to use these on a partner, take a class! Watch online and in-person demonstrations. (See examples in Figure 4-9.)

- **Canes:** Rattan and bamboo are favored woods for caning, with rattan being more flexible and bamboo more rigid. If you are a kinkster who wants a heavier hit with your cane, materials like fiberglass or aluminum are for you. If you want to maximize flexibility and smoothness of stroke, rattan is best. Thinner canes sting worse.

>> **Punching, hitting, slapping:** Like spanking, during a punching, hitting or slapping scene, it's important to be able to monitor the impacted area. If you are striking the face, a best practice is to hold onto the chin so that you minimize impact on the head. Never backhand. It may seem like slapping doesn't require training, but if you are hitting or slapping the face or head, you need it.

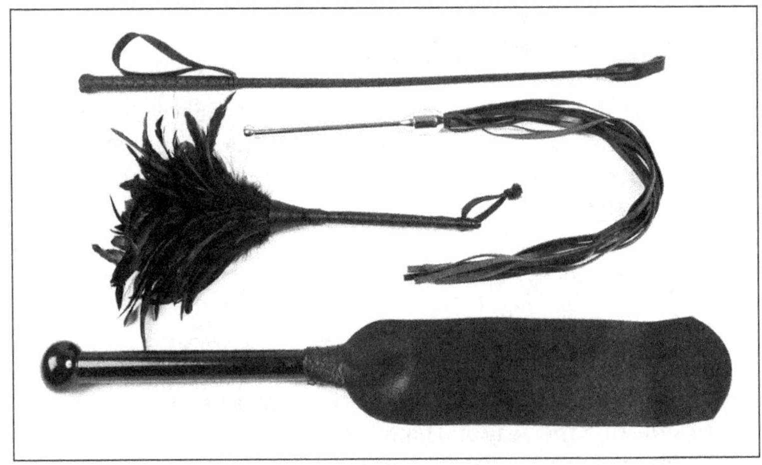

FIGURE 4-9: Assorted whips and paddles.

© der_bilstein/Adobe Stock Photos

> **»** **Flogging:** Braided leather floggers are most beloved for flogging scenes, but they come in all kinds of materials, like pleather, paracord or rope. Flexible and soft materials that are wider are "thuddy" floggers while stiffer and shorter cutouts or "tails" create a "stinging" experience. The stiffer the tail, the more intense the sting.
>
> If you want to flog someone, take a class. *Take several.* Good flogging technique protects your arm and serves your partners. A best practice for flogging is to change-up the target area of your impact periodically and move your hands over the affected areas to assess and soothe as you go.

TIP

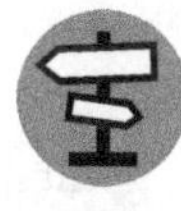

KINK
STORY

At one play party, I watched a Top punch a bottom multiple times in the chest. Sometimes upper chest, above the breasts and sometimes actually on the breasts. He hit her so hard! At the time I was extremely uncomfortable and thought, "HELL NO! This is not for me. Neither as a Top nor as a bottom." But a few years later, I began to feel curious about this act. First, I punched a few people, and that was fun! Then, I asked a trusted partner to give me a few hits on the upper chest. To my shock, it felt good, almost like a massage. I still do not like it at all on my breasts, but I do enjoy it on my upper chest. Recently another play partner had tied my hands together up above my head and was punching my chest. I was like, "OW! This doesn't feel good!" They said, "here, let's untie your hands so you can put them down. That changes the sensation." Once we did that, it was back to the enjoyable feeling that I was seeking in that moment. —**Robin**

Hot wax and fire play

Second only to the connection between the players, great hot wax play is all about the materials. Many kinksters love the ritual of heating the wax. You may love the anticipation — the build-up, the change-up, the intense sensations, and the wheres and whens of hot wax in a scene. Kinksters report feeling cared for and aroused by the attention playing with wax requires.

Similarly, fire play involves using fire close to or directly on the skin. This can arouse fear and spike your adrenaline. It can also cause a range of sensations from the mild feeling of heat akin to hot, to significant pain. For some kinksters, fire taps into a primordial symbolism or can remind them of learning about the power of fire as a child. Fire play is often combined with ritual dance or other celebrations.

WARNING

Be sure you are using wax that melts at a lower temperature, such as soy or paraffin wax. Don't use beeswax, microcrystalline, or stearin wax. Be aware that dyes can raise a melting point, while mineral oil can lower it. Check the condition of you and your partners' skin periodically. Think about how allergies might play out.

If you are playing with fire, always have a fire blanket; extinguisher; wet cloths; Kevlar-coated, fire-safe toys and tools; moisturizer; and a first aid kit that includes burn gel on hand. And observers/spotters should be nearby.

Needless to say, hot wax and fire play are not for beginners. If you are interested in this type of play, observe, take classes, and find experienced practitioners to learn from.

Taking great care of your materials and safety gear is essential to enjoying the many pleasures of hot wax and fire.

Genital pain play and pleasure denial

It's hard to think of a more vulnerable site of pain play than your genitals. Cock and ball torture (CBT), chastity play, clit and labia clamping, piercings, and sounding are examples of genital pain play. CBT can include compression, tying up, piercing, hitting, or stomping on the penis or balls (ball busting). Chastity play may include using cock cages or chastity belts to lock up the genitals of the sub, sometimes painfully, for the Dom's exclusive authority or use. Clit and labia clamps and piercings take advantage of the tremendous number of nerve endings on the clitoris and the tenderness and vulnerability of the labia to create a pain/pleasure experience. And *sounding* involves the careful insertion of rods into the penis and urethra to create a highly vulnerable and pleasurable shared outcome. If your kink fantasies revolve around the vulnerability, sluttiness, amazingness, imagined shortcomings, or responsiveness of your genitals — this kind of play may be for you.

Play piercing

Play piercing most often involves multiple superficial piercings of the skin, perhaps in specific patterns, to bring on endorphin rushes for the players. Kinksters describe their experiences of ritual piercings as erotically or spiritually charged, often leaving temporary or permanent scarring, depending on the desires of the players involved. Unlike a blood draw, play piercing involves the needle passing through rather than into the skin, so that both ends are visible. Play piercing itself can sometimes bring its recipients to orgasm.

A kinkster may prefer more intense piercing play, involving heavier hooks from which they may be suspended by their play partners.

Hook suspension piercing is peak level piercing scenario only for advanced players who have access to highly trained teammates. By piercing the skin with hooks and suspending the player, many kinksters often pass through a kind of spiritual portal to healing and change.

This is a category of play that requires a lot of training and trust, including attention to the sterilization of all materials, which is a must in any piercing play.

Microbranding or tattooing

Some kinksters desire permanent marking of their bodies during play, with many describing this as spiritual or a part of how they celebrate their culture or identity. Many people who have extensive or all-body tattoos describe the protracted experience of being tattooed as trance-inducing, a peak kink experience; and the relationship between them and their tattoo artist as singular. Consciously kink-identified tattoo artists are in great demand and have a legacy of kink play and artistry that one can track through a kink community.

Microbranding or cell-popping is less common than tattooing and involves the use of cautery pens to draw designs on a sub. Both tattooing and branding require significant training in the both the practice of creating the art and attention to aftercare. If you are looking for a partner to tattoo or brand you, check out their work and their aftercare reputation.

Unless you have very significant funding to correct them, any branding and extensive tattooing create permanent body alterations. Be certain about your desire and your partners if you are seeking brands or tattoos. And if you want to take on these practices, look for people whose practices you love and admire in finding your training options.

Psychological play

An intense S/M arena involves psychological play, with interrogation scenes and military or policing scenes being prized. These often draw in other kinds of S/M play. Our contributor Naria notes that this is a favored practice for them:

> One of my favorite types of play is hardcore interrogation — police or military style. It's immersive, high-intensity role-play built around a storyline, but the scene itself is both physically and psychologically demanding. I especially enjoy pushing the "prisoner" or "person of interest" to their limits to "break" them and extract the information I'm after. I use a range of implements — canes, batons, single tails, even punching — combined with stress positions and constant in-character intensity. Interrogation play is a brutal, strategic dance of endurance, control, and mind games. And while it's rough and raw, it can also be incredibly freeing — and even healing.

Sadists have to wade through a lot of stigma and negativity to claim and explore their kinks. This is partly because the moniker *sadism* comes from the practices of the Marquis De Sade, who does not meet the qualification of a kinkster in this book because all of the practices here hinge on consent. De Sade, by contrast, was instead a dangerous and unrelenting abuser.

Masochists also carry a heavy stigma burden from the passing commentators of the disdaining world. Like their sadistic counterparts, masochists are often judged as "sick" with a particular bent on self-destruction.

I tire of the damning eyes of others on your fantastical kinky aspirations. Somewhere around my late 40s, I got so tired that I actually don't think about them anymore. Writing this book has reminded me of how overwhelming and intrusive those gawping eyes (and yapping jaws) can be.

I feel fortunate to have been raised in queer community, where the powerful advice of Stonewall veteran and trans activist Marsha P. Johnson rules. Marsha said that the P. in her name stood for *Pay It No Mind*. Accordingly, your best response to someone who implies that your S/M desires make you a sad victim or a monster is to live your best, ecstatic kinky life — to cherish and care for your play partners and lovers, and to take phenomenal care of yourself. And to the buzz-killing, omnipresent eye: *Pay It No Mind*.
—Jaime

Safety basics for S/M

Safety specifics of S/M track with the safety directions in other kink categories:

>> Pay attention to your emotional condition.

>> Pay attention to your physical condition.

>> Check your props and materials: fabric, sterilization, proper wax, and so on.

>> Know that the quality of the intimate exchange is key.

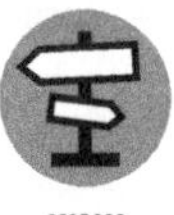

KINK STORY

Years ago, I coined my own kink: Compression Play. It's sadistic deep-tissue massage meets sensual dominance. Less about strikes — more about weight. Pressure. Slowness. A finger becomes a drill. A knuckle, an anchor. I press into pressure points with full presence, eyes locked. It's bodywork meets power exchange. Submission through kneading. I roll them, dig in, use my full body weight to claim space on and inside them. The stretch. The grind. The unbearable fullness of being pressed into surrender. There's no flurry of movement — only slow, controlled force. Breath and pressure, muscle and command. It's intimate and intense. I give it. I crave it. It bypasses pain and slips straight into catharsis. It's not just impact — it's immersion. **—Ignacio**

Setting Up Role-Play and Fantasy

For some kinksters, role-play and fantasy play are the ultimate kink avenues. As a role player, the important thing for you may be creating distance between your real life and the character you play. You may need definitive lines between yourself and the specific temperament or core actions of the character or the outrageousness or intensity of the scenario you've created.

TIP

If, as many kinksters say, the sexiest organ in the body is the brain, there's perhaps no better place in kinky life to stretch that sexy organ than role-play. Because your kinky mind is capable of endless creation, there is literally no end to the possibilities.

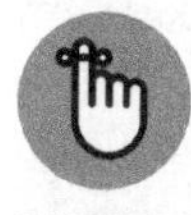

REMEMBER

Indeed, role-play lives in all of the other domains of kink mentioned in this chapter. Because if you are a D/s enthusiast, you might not see yourself as a role player, but you are taking on a role, like Mommy or Daddy. If you are a committed sadist or masochist — same. You are putting yourself into a role that gratifies you, and in doing so, stepping into the heightened arena of intimate play.

But role players in kink life go even further. They make up specific kink scenarios that heighten their pleasure. Some engage in elaborate scripting, costuming, and/or creation of the scene for their play.

Age and age-gap play

Age play involves reverting to a younger persona in your play and finding others who share this interest. "Littles" enjoy the freedom of childhood or babyhood in their scenes. Littles may have Tops who chaperone their play with other littles and keep them safe.

Age-gap play, sometimes referred to as "dark" age play, is more controversial. People who love age-gap play can go all the way to an infantile state, which hands over maximal control to their older play partners, or they can play with youth-adult scenarios, which enters a highly taboo area of play.

Age-gap play is an arena of play that various police forces may track because there are a lot of violent, harmful practices happening daily — enacted by abusive people who are doing the opposite of what kinksters do. *They are harming young people.*

If you love age play, protect yourself. Play in online spaces that are encrypted or in kink environments that are long-standing and well-managed for your safety, and the well-being of everyone involved.

Breeding, pregnancy, breastfeeding, milking

Many people associate intense feelings with pregnancy, whether it's a desire to have a baby, fear of unwanted pregnancy, or the high-stakes commitment to another a person through the decision to become pregnant. This source of intensities becomes the stuff of play when kinksters draw upon it to create a scene.

There are so many ways to play in this territory. Kinksters love Mommy play and the vulnerability and connection of breastfeeding. You may love playing with the theatrical complexities of pregnancy. You may be interested to play with gender around who is impregnating or breastfeeding from whom. As with so many aspects of role-play, one's actual embodiment is just a point of departure for the endless possibilities of fantasy.

Furries

Furries are people with an interest in characters portrayed with a mix of animal and human characteristics. Many furries create personas, or fursonas, for themselves as a role-play character. For some, their fursona becomes a deeply-held aspect of their identity.

Many furries are happy role-playing in a fun and non-sexual way and that fully satisfies their desire. For others, they may role-play online or consume furry-themed pornography but never really take their fursona into sexual spaces in real life. And for still others, they may fully act out and embody their characters during sex.

Fur suits, costumes that allow furries to inhabit their fursona in physical space, can be as elaborate as sports team mascots or as minimal as ears on a headband or a tail coming out of a belt. For many furries, two big considerations around "suiting up" are the cost of the costume and heat exhaustion. Full custom fur suits in the manner of a mascot cost a lot and are thus financially inaccessible to many. In terms of comfort, heavy fur can easily cause a kinkster to overheat during play, so intense scenes and high exertion sex might not work in full costume.

Pet play: puppies and ponies

Pet play has been around for a very long time but it's come into light more in our current era of social media. Similar to furries, many pet players may create a persona, determining what kind of animal they want to play as well as a name (many pups use names that incorporate the word pup like Pup Onyx or Stray Pup) but also what temperament they want to take on and how easily they can be controlled by a partner.

A common form of equipment for pup play is a black leather hood that evokes the features of a dog. Some pup hoods may also be fuzzy or furry. Pups also often wear tails that attach belts or to butt plugs that may remain in place during play. Ponies also adopt costumes that bring them closer to their animal counterparts, like hooves. They may wear bit gags, enjoy being secured as a work horse to a wagon, and invite being whipped in the manner of a horse.

As with other forms of role-play, pups and ponies draw misunderstanding from uninitiated onlookers who may assume that players are interested in bestiality, rather than inhabiting a role where they offer the services and pleasures of a pet or working animal. Pets love letting go of the obligations of having a fully functional human brain and full faculties of communication, allowing them to access different forms of domination and submission and also different forms of love and affection.

Universal role-play

Role players love the theater of play. They are aroused by the great lengths their imaginations go to in setting scenes and playing out all kind of possible intimate connections. Three key aspects of role-play that stretch your imagination are described in this section.

Dressing for the part

For many role players, everything happens in the mind and no physical symbolic markers are necessary or desired. But for some, dressing the part shifts their brains into a new persona or into the intimate space of the scene. For still others, the outfits themselves may be the most compelling part of the kink.

When co-creating a scene with someone, talking beforehand about what kind of clothes you see yourself in can be a powerful way to communicate about your desire. In fact, whether you're able to create the exact outfit that's in your mind, talking about the scene may help your partners to better grasp the character and experience you're imagining. Kinksters all over the world have found ways to evoke a look through even small pieces of clothing. Get creative and communicate!

Setting the stage and getting started

If you love developing scenes in your mind, you might love elaborate staging for your scenes. Some kinksters will transform their basements or apartments for a desired role-play. Or you may like to scout locations for public scenes that you choreograph privately. Find that smokey bar of your dreams for a pick-up scene. Locate a beautiful cruising area. Pick an iconic location that has a formal meaning (hello, Washington Monument) and transform it with your kinky script.

When we suggest role-play to people who aren't experienced, the number one thing they mention as being a point of anxiety is how to start. There's no one-size-fits-all way to set the stage for a scene. It can be fun to start role-playing as soon as someone comes through the door. Some kinksters like to establish a small ritual that signals the start of a scene, like sitting down, breathing deeply together, or lighting a candle. If you are nervous, you may want to start kissing and touching first, and then once you and your scene partners are in a state of arousal, one person may whisper something in the other's ear — in character — to signal the start of the role-play.

Safety basics for role-play

This section provides a few key basics to consider for diving into role-play safely.

Falling down the rabbit hole

It can be helpful to have a sense of how deep you and your partners are into the specific aspects of your roles before getting into it. The stakes are higher for this kind of play if your role touches on raw areas of your life experience or your partner's. For example, two survivors of violence may be playing with violent personas or characters, but one may want to lean into intense details that may not work for the other.

Beyond issues of role-playing with violence, getting into character and playing for long periods can be emotionally demanding. Pay attention to how far into your character you've fallen, and how well your partner is faring in the scenes. Sometimes, your intense attachment to the role can be more taxing than you realize. Stay grounded and alert to your physical and emotional condition.

Grounding practices

Having a good grounding practice is crucial in any kinkster's life and will be very useful to you when delving into role-play. If you feel yourself losing the thread between you and your character so that you no longer can track the boundaries you've agreed to in a scene, you may need to take a time-out.

Kinksters draw on all kinds of practices to stay grounded. Kinkster Anna Meyer has a somatics method (see Appendix A) for quick grounding if you feel yourself beginning to fray — from stomping your feet to remind yourself where you are, to rubbing your chest between your clavicles to center comfort and move any frozen energy in your chest, to breathing deeply over several breaths to help you gain clarity in the moment. Any of these techniques will help ground you in who you are and what the limits of consent are in this scenario.

Role-playing can generate massive endorphin rushes, and staying grounded will allow you to pursue your kinky joy with abandon.

Be careful what you record

We've mentioned throughout the book that not everything that makes sense to you as a kinkster in a scene will make sense to an outsider. As long as you are grounded in consent and mutual respect, you can free yourself of others' judgment. But be careful when creating any kind of digital trail or record that may extend beyond that scene. Kinky in-character texts leading up to a scene, for example, may be discoverable by others and can expose you in ways that can harm you in your family or public life. If you're playing with intense themes like age gaps, devastation, and CNC — often the very things that kinksters draw upon to heal or to amplify arousal — it can be misinterpreted and misconstrued by outsiders. Be smart and self-protective about your kink records.

Investigating Leather

Some kinksters relate to their kinky sexuality and practices as the drivers of their community-building and family life. Nowhere is this more evident or thoughtfully constructed than among Leather kinksters and in Leather communities.

Leather subculture

The Leather subculture is rooted in visual props and cues, which involve a lot of leather, but it's more than that as well. Common garments include harnesses, cuffs, vests, chaps, hats, leather pants, and jackets. While many of these items are made of leather, other materials can be in the mix including denim, rubber, and spandex. These days there are even Leather community members who refuse to wear leather for reasons pertaining to animal rights or environmental sustainability. These kinksters opt for faux leather with no animal involvement.

The Leather subculture is steeped in symbolism, often drawing on symbols of masculinity from non-kinky culture but using them in novel ways. For example, many common leather garments reference military garb, like a garrison hat or military-style boots. These authoritarian symbols are used by the Leather community, prioritizing consent, pleasure, and community care rather than literal aggression or an impulse to conquer.

Another way in which the Leather community draws on the symbolism is the highly developed color palette. While the most common color for leather items is black, there are many other colors that can communicate a lot to other community members. Yellow piping on a leather harness, for example, may indicate an interest in watersports, and wearing a lot of red may mean the person is into fisting. (These kinks are discussed later in this chapter.)

Color-coded communication

The most famous example of this kind of color-coded communication is the "hanky code," which originated with Leather men but has been also across many communities, notably among queers. Placing a handkerchief in the back left pocket, or anywhere on the left side of the body, generally means the person is a Top; the right side denotes bottom. And the color indicates the particular kink the person is interested in pursuing as Top or bottom (see Table 4-1).

TABLE 4-1

Hanky Codes

Color	Meaning
White	Mutual masturbation
Light blue	Oral sex
Navy blue	Anal sex
Teal blue	Co** and ball torture
Red	Fisting
Magenta	Piercing
Purple	Armpit worship
Gray	Bondage

Color	Meaning
Black	SM
Hunter green	Daddy play
Yellow	Piss
Brown	Scat
Beige	Rimming
Fuchsia	Spanking
Coral	Foot worship

Formal practices, relationships, and traditions

Being in the Leather scene holds different meaning for kinksters. For some, it might mean that they like the clothing style or they like the vibe at Leather bars. For many, it includes a focus on formalized roles in kinky play and creating networks of people who teach one another how to fulfill their desires with a sense of tradition, mastery, and empowerment. The community has a deep commitment to mentorship, ensuring that each generation of Leather practitioners passes on their wisdom and expertise so that Leather players feel well-prepared to build their kinky lives.

Leather families

Many Leather people build relationships more enduring than simply being involved in a loose community of kinksters — by forming Leather families. As with other forms of BDSM community, there's often a focus on hierarchy and service, with patriarchs and/or matriarchs sitting atop of a family tree and various relations cascading down through mentorship, teaching, shared rituals, love, sex, kink, and devotion that can last a lifetime.

For LGBTQ+ people and others who have experienced life as "outsiders" on some level, Leather families can create a replacement for their families of origin that may have been disrupted by rejection, with religious dogma, sexism, homophobia, and transphobia being the common drivers for being cast out. But even those Leather people who maintain relationships with their extended families may find deep meaning and familial fulfillment in Leather relationships. In particular, the structure and hierarchy it provides can help kinksters feel secure about their exploration of kink within a community of loved ones. In this way, Leather practitioners and families form a circle of care around their beloveds.

Jack, for example, has a Leather Daddy who has offered nurturing and mentorship as an older activist with similar interests. For him, having a Daddy isn't like having a boyfriend or a husband; it is a unique form of relating that has grown out of Leather culture and has allowed him to access kinky places of vulnerability that is reserved just for this special relationship.

Shaan, another contributor, is an accomplished bootblack. Bootblacks champion service and take on the crucial role of caring for leather boots and other leather pieces such as jackets and harnesses. The importance of the bootblack role in the community is evident in its centrality to Leather contests around the world, where practitioners demonstrate their skills and fiercely compete for the title of Best Bootblack.

Leather leaders in the fight against AIDS

As an extension of that circle of care, Leather communities have played a crucial part in responding and fighting to end the HIV/AIDS epidemic. Innumerable Leather people lost their lives as part of the epidemic, and the community responded powerfully by leaning into their strengths as sex educators, helping people learn about and avoid transmission of the virus.

Many community events, such as the Leather contests and club runs, were made into fundraisers for HIV/AIDS research and advocacy. Through these efforts, millions and millions of dollars for community-based care have been raised over the past nearly half century.

LEATHER CLUBS

Leather culture first appeared among gay and bi men following World War II, with major early centers of Leather life in California, though today's Leather communities encompass all genders, sexualities, and geographies.

Leather Clubs were an early way that gay Leather men created space for themselves to commune and practice kink. In the 1950s, gay motorcycle clubs like the Satyrs Motorcycle Club and Oedipus Motorcycle Club, both in Los Angeles, were established and patterned after straight biker clubs. These groups created community connection for men who sought kink and relational spaces that weren't open to the general public and allowed them to feel safe at a time when their sexuality was particularly stigmatized and criminalized.

Surveying Other Kinky Possibilities

As noted in the chapter's intro, it's difficult to provide a complete list of kinks because they're endless. You can have an amplified or kinky attachment to literally anything: candles, rose petals, a smell, your car, lip piercings, a celebrity, a fictional character. Anything you encounter or experience can potentially generate a heightened response — whether an intensely sexualized or highly vulnerable state — thus creating a potential kink.

In the previous sections, we've gone over some classic, established kink categories. Here are some others that are immensely popular among kinksters, but perhaps less commonly discussed beyond the scene.

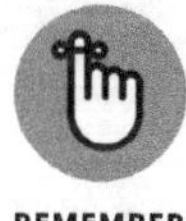

REMEMBER

If you have an out-of-the-box kink and you think nobody else in the world has it, think again.

Party or group scenes and dungeon play

Group scenesters love a play party, a circle jerk, an orgy, a bathhouse, a sex club, a dungeon or any other opportunity to have or observe sex communally. If your kink fantasies revolve around groups, there are many different settings to observe or try out your kink. Online spaces like Fetlife (see Appendix B) can point you to local opportunities or events you can travel to if you'd prefer to be anonymous or out of town to try out your enthusiasm for group or party sex.

You may want to do an assessment of the people you could theoretically run into in a group or semipublic sex space and have a plan for how you would handle the situation if you saw the wrong person. For example, if you show up at a sex club and you see a coworker who you supervise, your plan might be to turn around and walk out of the club.

A specific type of group play many kinksters enjoy is dungeon play. Dungeons are generally private membership clubs that are fully stocked with toys and equipment to help you act out the scenes you dream of. This may include smaller pieces like whips and floggers. It can also include furniture-sized equipment like sex slings or a *Saint Andrew's Cross,* an x-shaped cross a sub can be strapped to with their legs spread and immobilized to receive discipline (see Figure 4-10).

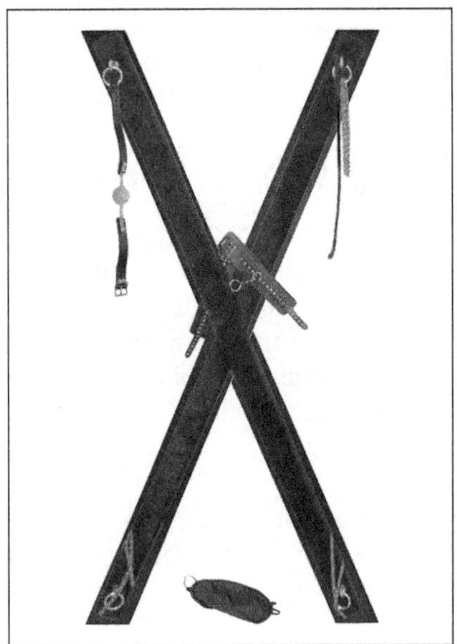

FIGURE 4-10: A typical Saint Andrew's Cross.

© JFsPic/Adobe Stock Photos

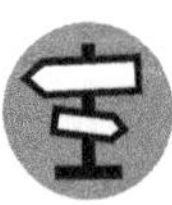

I once went through an eyebrow-plucking phase — mirror, tweezers, precision. I didn't know then that what thrilled me wasn't beauty — it was *extraction* (the act of pulling something out). One night at a dungeon, a pair of tweezers fell from our bag mid-scene. My lover picked them up instinctively and began plucking. Me — bound to the St. Andrew's Cross. Legs apart. Still. One pull at a time. Every hair a jolt of pain-pleasure. That moment cracked something open. Now, it's tweezers and wax: genitals, buttholes, toes — anywhere. A little sadism. A little artistry. Erotic extraction. Like a Dr. Pimple Popper clip . . . but filthy, slow, deliberate. And hot as hell. I love giving it. I love receiving it. I love the ritual of it. Precision as power. **—Ignacio**

For many kinksters, dungeon play isn't just about the furniture or the club, it's about access to an expansive, shared kink experience in community. You may find dungeon play to be a place of liberation that is unlike any other space in your life. It may mean access to a space where you can meet friends, potential playmates, and even partners. And if you want the social aspects and the use of equipment but group play isn't your thing, some dungeons have private areas that can be reserved.

Feet and other body fetishes

Feet are a common fixation for kinksters, but any body part can become someone's kink or fetish. For some, it's about having your own feet touched, massaged, or kissed; for others, it's all about worshipping your partners' feet or catching a glimpse of other people's feet in open-toed shoes. Conversely, your foot fetish may leave the world of worship altogether and be a favorite place on the body to inflict or enjoy pain.

Other common body-part kinks include hands and armpits. But you can also have a fetish for parts of the body that are so commonly discussed as amplifiers of arousal that most people wouldn't even see them as a kink — like a fixation on breasts or butts.

Fisting

Inserting your whole fist into a person's vagina or butt or having their fist inside you can be among the most intense and intimate ways of bonding with another person. Depending on a number of factors, it can involve a lengthy period of stretching with fingers and toys, building up to the moment of full fist penetration.

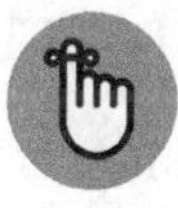

REMEMBER

Fisting a vagina or a butt are very different processes. The vaginal opening is more elastic, stretching more easily than anal tissue, but the rectum has more depth and can often accept further intrusion, well past the wrist. Patience is a virtue, and lube is your best friend, in either case. Use non-oil-based lubes for the vagina, oil-based lubes for the butt.

TIP

Many fisters homebrew their own lubricants to maximally reduce friction and increase safety and pleasure. Many also use nitrile gloves to minimize the potential for creating cuts with your nails, and possible allergic reactions.

You shouldn't experience painful rubbing sensations during the fisting experience. If that isn't the case, you may need to stop the scene and try a different fisting approach, and possibly different lube formulation.

If you or your partners have a history of vaginal spasms or pain, or ruptured hemorrhoids, be careful with fisting, as this could cause medical complications.

Blood play and medical scenes

Blood play describes practices that involve drawing or using blood in a kink scene or encounter. It often entails cutting with knives or other implements and can include menstrual blood. Blood can be drawn from very hard flogging as well, or kinksters may use blood that is produced from an incidental injury.

Blood play is among the kinks that require you to be fully informed about the health risks of bodily fluid exchange. It also requires sterilized surgical instruments, never common knives, and entails communicating with partners about health issues like HIV status, knowing where on the body is safest for play, and keeping emergency supplies nearby.

For some, blood scenes could be a part of a role-play involving vampires or medical personnel. For many, there's an intense association between drawing blood and being at the doctor's office. Doctors hold significant power with their patients because their extensive training prompts you to give them the power to make life or death decisions about your body. All of this intensity creates a well of energy that kinksters draw upon when creating medical scenes, whether they involve blood, costumes, or simple verbal role-play.

Electrostimulation

Some kinksters use electricity as a medium for scene play. Often called erotic electrostimulation (or e-stim for short), it involves stimulation of nerves with energy from a power source like a transcutaneous electrical nerve stimulation (TENS) unit.

A TENS unit is a small machine that produces mild electric current often used to fire nerves and muscles for therapeutic purposes, but that same mild current can be used to create more intense sensations and even pain.

Many kinksters apply e-stim to the genitals and then play with intensity levels, but this can be done anywhere on the body.

Watersports, spitting, and scat

Kinksters may use bodily fluids as both symbols and concrete representations in their play. Watersports refers to the use of urine for this purpose, and scat refers to human feces.

For some, these excretions can symbolize degradation and be the ultimate form of humiliation. Sharing or propelling your bodily fluids upon a partner can trip deep internal wiring that seeks to hide or dispose of our personal waste and avoid diseases, but going against the grain of that programming is exactly the thing that can make the play so cathartic and satisfying.

For other kinksters, spitting or scat play isn't symbolic at all. The way your desire works, you may simply respond joyously to the flavor of urine and revel in the intimacy of a partner sharing excretions with you. It may not be a symbol of degradation or humiliation at all, but a gift of the sacred.

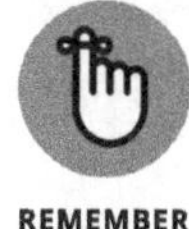

Don't yuck my (or another person's) yum. This is one of the few hard and fast rules of kink life. For kinksters into scat, for example, they are well aware of the majority consensus that this is gross. In fact, that revulsion may be connected to why they want it. You don't need to share your opinion about scat if you are in the majority. Similarly, when you're writing a dating app profile or a personal ad, it's best to discuss what you are into rather than offer any kind of judgmental language about what doesn't interest you.

Rubber and fetishwear

Kinksters who love rubber are often aroused by the feel, smell, texture of the material, and the *compression* (the feeling of being packed so tightly into a rubber outfit) that hugs all of your muscles and releases positive hormones.

In the same way that some people love rubber and some people love leather, a kinkster may fetishize any textile, material, or style. You may love a certain kind of period of clothing and build your fetish around it.

For example, "fifties housewife" is a favorite clothing and role-play fetish, digging deeply into pony skirts and pointy structured bras, as well as the gendered dynamics of 1950s suburban life. Cosplay can become part of a kink fetish, or the costumes in your favorite movie, from *Pirates of the Caribbean* to *The Birds*. Kinksters love reveling in their favorite aesthetics and drawing on these looks, fabrics, and ways of being in their scenes.

24/7 kink life

For a subset of kinksters, the time-limited kink scene doesn't satisfy their kink impulses, and they desire to take their play into their daily life, creating agreements with partners that don't end when a kink scene is over. These kinksters may be into 24/7, or a kink life that involves kink dynamics 24 hours a day, 7 days a week.

For some, this may mean setting up a surveillance system where a Dom has access to a Ring camera video feed, so they can see when their sub comes and goes from their house. For others, it means having the direct deposit of their wages go straight into a bank account from which their Dom can control daily financial transactions. Still others may set up a free use consent agreement so that they've agreed their partner can "force" them to have sex anytime they want (although the consent agreements often detail certain boundaries like not when guests are around).

For many, the encompassing nature of the 24/7 power exchange creates healthy and joyful ways of being.

It's important to note that this kind of dynamic also raises the stakes significantly on the potential for abuse.

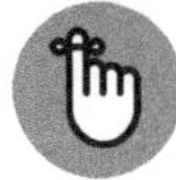

Someone having total control of your bank account, for example, means that if you need to break off the relationship, you are financially vulnerable and may have difficulty leaving. Also, being in a state of arousal or near-arousal 24/7 can be taxing, and it may take time for you to realize this or figure out what adjustments need to be made so that you feel more balanced.

Whether as a Dom or a sub, a 24/7 contract is an enormous expression of trust and a tremendous responsibility (see Chapter 8 for a sample contract.). Choose both the terms of your 24/7 agreement and your partners wisely.

Safety basics in less common kinks

If you find yourself exploring kinks that are less commonly discussed than others, not to worry, there are still many kinksters who share your passion for said object or practice. And, as is true for safety concerns in other, more common kinky lanes, strong safety basics will take care of you. Per usual:

>> Pay attention to yourself and your partners.

>> Check your gear — whatever you are into. You can find advice about it from kinksters who have helped create safer practices by using better materials.

>> Say what you mean, be who you say you are, keep your promises.

>> Treasure the space you are creating, the people you are creating it with, and yourself.

What time is it? Time to think more deeply about the feelings these various kink possibilities provoke. In Chapter 5, you can take all of these definitions and hypothetical play scenarios and throw them into the mix with your own desires and fantasy life.

2

Building Your Kinky Life

Chapter **5**

Discovering and Claiming Your Kinks

Kinsters find unique facets of themselves in the kinky scenarios and relationships they create. For many, kink provides the only portal to this kind of self-connection and expression. Kinksters describe being able to connect to their deepest desires through kink as singularly liberating and a crucial part of their inner life and sexuality.

In this chapter, you can undertake many activities to uncover and consider your kink desires and aspirations. We use inventories to help you track your experiences and consider where they may be pointing you on your path toward kink play. Your kinky truth is out there — or more precisely, *it's in there.*

Wherever you find yourself in your process, you deserve a fantastic, spicy, surprising, and gratifying lifelong journey with your kinks, where one discovery leads to another.

Letting Yourself Know What You Know

When it comes to kink and sexuality, it can be difficult to recognize and claim what you already know about yourself. You may have watched a movie or read a book and found yourself wildly turned on by something you've never considered an acceptable or appropriate way to relate to someone. You may have come upon a friend or family member engaged in an intimate exchange that shocked you. Many kinksters feel ambivalent about these revelatory moments and tell themselves that the lingering arousal or passion for this kind of connection was because it was a surprise or a taboo. You may have given yourself a million reasons to suppress a desire that has seemed out of bounds or impossible to express with another person.

TIP

There's a whole world of kink and lovely kinksters who have been where you are — in a state of self-discovery. You can make choices about your desire that are right for you.

Inventorying your intimate practices

A great way to begin this exploration is to just start where you are. You live in a culture that sells sex at every corner and discusses kink endlessly via social media, but spaces to be honest and vulnerable? *Very rare.* Let's make one for you right here, starting with some simple steps.

This following exercise is an expansion of Desire Mapping offered in Jaime's book, *Great Sex: Mapping Your Desire.* Here, we refer to it as a *desire inventory.*

>> **Set up a desire grid.** Draw a grid with four age markers — see the grid that follows as an example. Hypothetically, if you are 65 and have 50 years of sexuality and desire to map out, use 12-year markers. If you are 30 and have 15 years to map, use 3-year markers. You may want to label your markers so that they cover eras instead of years like: "College" or "Lived in NC." You get the idea. Create a spectrum with four era markers and seven subject-categories. A sample grid for a 35-year-old is shown in the table following this list.

> If you are a highly reflective person or experienced at journaling, your grid could take up a whole composition book. If you prefer visual art explorations, hang a grid on the wall and draw or paste in images that represent this period of your life. If simplicity is king, create a simple block grid and put two-word representations of the era into each box.

>> **Note your key fantasies.** These are scenarios you acted out in your mind during this era, when you were with someone or alone, that were

foundational to your desire and your pleasure. This may have emerged from something you read about, watched on TV or in porn, or observed.

>> **Write down your favorite thing or kink dynamic that arouses you.** Recall a *kink dynamic* (a real or imagined connection between you and another kinkster such as Daddy/girl or Owner/pup) that you returned to over and over in this era — this could be a flirtation, way of being, or sexual practice that was sure to get you going. These could be really different in each year marker, for example a kinkster may recall: Deep kissing made me hot at 15; I loved flogging masochists the most at 30.

>> **Write down your favorite sexual practice that brings you to orgasm.** Remember your favorite way of getting off in this era. If you do not seek or have orgasms, think of the number one practice that brings you the kind of pleasure or intimacy you seek. These can really shift across time. You might say: I loved double penetration in my 30s (see Appendix A); I loved solo sex with a vibrator in my 50s.

>> **Document your experience of the event.** Ask yourself: what was the way of being or feeling you longed for or experienced in this era or kink scene? How did the interaction impact you? What did you get? How would you describe yourself here?

>> **Describe the characteristics or roles of your lust subjects.** How would you best describe the subjects of your lust in this era? A kinkster may report: I loved people who were smaller than me in my teens and somewhat mean. In my 20s, I lusted after hairy dudes who treated me like a princess. In my 40s, I am hot for nonbinary partners whose genders and roles sometimes shift when we play.

>> **List your characteristics or roles.** Who are *you* in your kink and sexual intimacies in this era? Are you a tender care giver? A bossy director? A whiny submissive (sub)? A demanding slut? Remember your various personas and ways of being in this time period.

Kinksters may also describe how you carried yourself or dressed in each era: I loved cosplay and dressing up in my youth; and then in my 40s when I was parenting and had no time, I loved getting f*cked with nearly all our clothes on, fast and furious; now in my 50s, I enjoy formal dress at a fancy restaurant because it disguises how kinky I am.

>> **Share your favorite discovery about yourself in this period.** Turn your interpretive lens on yourself. Review. Ponder. What happened in this era that mattered? What did you learn about your desire? Kinksters may say: This was when I realized I liked watching others get off, or I liked being pushed until I cried, or I associated getting hit with orgasm.

Table 5-1 is a hypothetical grid for a 35-year-old kinkster.

TABLE 5-1   **Desire Inventory**

Desire Arena	Age 20	Age 25	Age 30	Age 35
Fantasy	Kissing against walls	Sex in the club	Lover comes home with friends	At a party, partner says: sit here
Kink dynamic	Being pushed or crowded	Many people are into me	Lover directs friends to f*ck me	Partner sends friends and strangers
Orgasmic: what gets me going/off	Slightly forced or coerced kissing	Group sex, feeling overwhelmed	Instrument of pleasure for others	I'm a public instrument of pleasure
My experience	Surprised, innocent	Surprised, unprepared	Shocked, obedient	Experienced sub, but the setting is a surprise
Characteristics/roles: them	Big, burly but with a heart of gold	Different kinds of hot men	Partner is a Dominant (Dom) of any gender	Dom and a voyeur, strict
Characteristics/roles: me	School girlish, ponytailed	Sexy, smart but didn't see this coming	Experienced, can provide pleasure	Sexy partygoer, love putting out for a Dom
Key discovery	Surprise, force, and naïveté are in the mix	Being overpowered is hot	Submitting to a Dom is pinnacle	I stretch to please my Dom

Examining your kink inventory

Inventories like the previous exercise can help you see what matters most in your desire and potential kink expression over time. They can help you discuss your history with potential partners and build more gratifying scenes. After you review your desire-grid responses, ask yourself the following questions:

>> What do you think about all of this?

>> How do you feel looking at it?

>> What has shifted the most over time?

>> Is there any desire or way of being that is fixed or a constant?

>> What's your grid telling you about you?

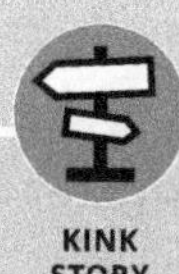

FIGURING IT OUT

In the early 90s, I was at a small house party mostly made up of friends I'd met through *Women in the Life*, in Washington, DC. Just like, maybe 10 to 12 people, getting together to play cards, cook/eat, talk — Be Black. Be queers hanging out.

And then, I don't know how it started to turn. But Truth or Dare was the catalyst. There were desire rumblings, but I didn't know all the connections; I was new. We're playing and the dares escalate because the sexual prowess–led shit talking starts to escalate, right? And as *that* escalates, we get to, *well, if you think you're such a badass, you can go down on me. Let's see you do x, y, and z.*

And I was like, is this really gonna happen? There was more trash talking, and then it happened! And my reaction was: *You know what? I don't mind. I don't mind this at all!* These were queer women, femmes, and Broads. Like — all my favorites. I mean, HELLO?!! So that's where I figured that kink out. Femmes with femmes and watching — CHECK. **—M'Bwende**

If you look at our fictional kinkster's responses in Table 5-1, the element of surprise is very important to her; it tracks across the 15-year period of her inventory. She starts out being aroused by her innocence and naiveté with someone who is in charge, but this morphs as she matures, and her expertise at giving pleasure becomes a sexy part of her kink. The genders of her partners change over time. Her ways of being are somewhat different across the years, but she could be described as consistently submissive. The temperament of her pushy crush or Dom moves from "heart of gold" in her youth to "strict" at her current age. You can't tell from this inventory whether the fantasy she describes lives only in her mind or has become part of what she co-creates with a Dom in person. She could use this inventory as a helpful starting place for conversations with potential playmates.

Determining what's missing

A great exercise to undertake in your desire and kink discovery process is to ponder what you've left out. When we present the Desire Mapping workshop at human rights conferences, a universal commonality across language and different cultures is that "Mappers" often suppress and deny parts of their history of arousal and desire out of fear or shame.

A difficulty many kinksters encounter in exploring and owning their kinks is that their play appears to contradict their identity or values. A Dom who believes in equality and highly respects the women in his life struggles with his desire to overpower and control his partners. A sub who has worked hard to battle discrimination and become a manager at work is ashamed of their passion for bottoming or humiliation. A hypermasculine athlete is terrified by his love of wearing feminine fetish gear. A person who champions openness and transparency is hiding her deep desire to be a kinky (consensual) stalker or voyeur.

Destructive or problematic power plays in the world plus desires that clash with your identity or values often combine to equal a favored kink.

It's your commitment to consent — the kink construct of play — that neutralizes all of these seemingly problematic desires.

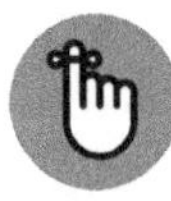

As long as you do no harm to yourself or any of your partners, your sexual and intimate life can pursue infinite, contradictory desire pathways, to the astonishment and joy of all involved.

Nothing has to make sense or add up. The art of kink sexuality is more like a chaotic Jackson Pollock painting than a precise rendering of the Dutch artist Rembrandt. You are rooting around in your illogical and disorderly wildness.

If you are wondering why your sexy or intimate encounters aren't really working for you, you may be suppressing important pieces of your desire puzzle. The following reflection questions may help you put it together:

>> What am I denying or minimizing about my desire that's important to me?

>> When did I start doing this?

>> Did an authority figure or system of authority shame me about this desire? What happened?

>> Is this figure or system of authority trustworthy? Have they harmed me in other ways?

Finish up your reflection with these concluding questions:

>> What might my intimate life be like if I claimed this desire and acted on it?

>> How would my sexual and relational life be different?

Let's go back to our fictional kinkster and see what she has to say when she adds a column to her inventory to list her hidden desires as shown in Table 5-2:

A Desire Inventory with Hidden Desires

	Age 20	Age 25	Age 30	Age 35	*Hiding*
Fantasy	Kissing against walls	Sex in the club	In my bed, lover comes home with friends	At a party, partner directs me to sit	Slap me across the face
Kink dynamic	Being pushed or crowded	Many people are into me	Lover directs friends to f*ck me	Partner sends friends and strangers to me	Humiliation
Orgasmic: what gets me going/off	Slightly forced or coerced kissing	Group sex, feeling overwhelmed	Instrument of pleasure for others	Public instrument of pleasure	"Corrected" by my Dom in public
My experience	Surprised, innocent	Surprised, unprepared	Shocked, obedient	Experienced sub, but the setting is a surprise	Shocked, ashamed, pitiful
Characteristics/ roles: them	Big, burly but heart of gold	Different kinds of hot men	Partner is a Dom of any gender, in charge	Dom and a voyeur, strict	Harsh disciplinarian Dom
Characteristics/ roles: me	School girlish, pony-tailed	Sexy, smart but didn't see this coming	Experienced, can provide pleasure	Sexy partygoer, love putting out for Dom	Bad Girl, a disappointment
Key discovery	Surprise, force, and innocence are the mix	Surprise, being overpowered is hot	Submitting to Dom is pinnacle	I want to stretch to meet Dom's desires	I want to play with disapproval and punishment in public

It's possible that our fictional sub lived with a lot of disapproval as a young person and managed this by overperforming. Maybe she organized her life to avoid physical punishment. Maybe she saw a slap in a movie when she was 10 and got wildly aroused but buried this desire. Or maybe she just wants to try this out and has been fearful around how much she wants it or hasn't found the right Dom to experiment with. Putting this desire on the grid takes the kink out from behind a curtain of shame and puts it on the table for her to consider, or at least to play with more in her fantasy life.

TIP

You can do it. You can tell yourself the thing you're hiding. You're in charge of how you play with your desire.

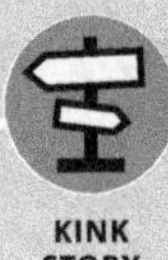

HOW CAN THESE TWO SIDES COEXIST?

As a therapist, I focus on providing support, intimacy, and gentleness for my clients. However, in my kink life, I often take on the role of a Dominant and find fulfillment in providing pain through *impact play* — typically spanking, paddling, and flogging.

At first, I couldn't understand how these two sides of me could coexist. I also dealt with some shame and confusion — how could my desires align with the values I hold as a therapist?

But after a lot of reflection, I've come to realize that these two roles aren't as contradictory as they seem. Both in my professional and kink life, consent, communication, and trust are key. In kink, I empower my partners by allowing them to surrender power to me, which is a form of trust and connection, rather than providing emotional support as I do in my daily life.

That sting I feel in the palm of my hand after I've just spanked my partner isn't about harm — I'm still offering care and support, but in a different way. **—Bishop**

Releasing shame and embracing contradiction

Despite what various authorities have told you about your unworthiness as a person or about the "inappropriateness" of your desire, you're still here. Still a desiring and desirable being. These next two activities are designed to help you reject shameful judgments about your kink sexuality.

THROWING OFF SHAME. Here's a favorite activity for exorcising shame. It's simple and effective. We highly recommend it.

1. **Pick up a ball, pillow, or orb of some kind.**

2. **Write a description of your shame on the object or the source of it (or both).** Alternatively, write your descriptions on pieces of paper and stuff them inside your pillow or mark the object in some way that denotes how you feel.

3. **Create an *impact play* experience.** Whack the object with your hands or knock the object against an immovable object, like a wall. You can use a racquet or anything that works besides your hand.

4. **Continue Step 3 while screaming one of the following suggestions.** (If you can't get privacy, scream in your head.)

- A *F*** You!* to the person who instilled the shame

- A strong "No" to reject the shame

- A directive to the shame — *F*** Off! Not today!*

- Any vocalization that feels freeing

5. **Repeat Steps 3 and 4 until you have completely exhausted yourself physically, vocally, and/or emotionally.**

   If you are with a supporter who loves and cares about you, which is recommended, give them the object to dispose of while you close out your experience of letting go. If you are solo, dispose as you wish.

6. **Breathe.** Take your time settling back into the present, and coming back to yourself.

7. **Re-connect to the present and your surroundings.** Make (or have your support person make) a celebratory beverage.

8. **Bring your beverage to sip in a comfortable setting.** Suggestions include your bed, your favorite chair, or any other incredibly comforting spot as you congratulate yourself and recoup.

Playing with complexity

As you consider whether you can handle the complexity and contradictions embedded in kink play, you may ask yourself: where else in my life do I manage and address complexity? If you're like us, the answer is: *everywhere.*

» As a friend, you may have a bestie who does not understand reciprocity. They may be draining, often demanding the center of attention. You may be frustrated by the amount of energy they take up, without noticing.

» As a parent, you may be ambivalent about being too strict or too open-minded with your child. You may tether back and forth. You may exhaust yourself in daily conflicts around getting to school on time or cleaning up after playtime. It may all seem so messy and trying at times.

» As a coworker, you may struggle with a work partner who always delivers late or can't stay on task, so you end up having to work overtime to make up for it. You may move between being overly affirming to try to point your coworker in the right direction and having meetings to convey your distress and your need for better, more timely outcomes.

All of these situations are actually struggles with power and honesty. They are navigations with the limits of time and patience and your desire to connect with people you deeply care about.

You play with these complexities all day long. You struggle with your values. You change course, you try new things.

Kink complexity is just like this. The muscles you exercise in your daily work and familial scenarios can be drawn upon to support you in navigating your kink scenarios. You can ask yourself:

>> Where is the power?

>> How do you want to enact or relinquish it?

>> What kind of time and energy do you have to put into a scene or a relationship?

>> Can you create something simple because life is demanding and time is short?

>> Have you found a true partner, or is this more of a one-time thing?

>> Can you really expose your most vulnerable kink longings, or is this connection more like kink-light?

In your daily life, you've cultivated a highly developed set of skills for getting through the complex demands of your day. Draw on these as you create pathways to your kink needs and wants. And, if you find that you're overwhelmed, you can work on improving on or building new relational skills (see Chapters 7 through 9).

Giving yourself permission

Sometimes you may find yourself waiting for others to give you the thing you must give yourself. This is a common occurrence in kink life, where you might seek the approval of friends or a lover or an important confidante or healer. You might think to yourself: if only X could understand and affirm my way of being or desire for this activity I want to pursue, then I could move forward.

But here's the thing: *You are X.*

You are the one who is holding you back. Your judgment of your desires, your belief that kink intimacy doesn't matter, or that if you fixed something about yourself, this longing or way of being would evaporate.

Of course, it's possible for you to have a happy life without kink. But why would you? Why choose to deny yourself these feelings and this mode of intimate connection when it keeps circling back to you again and again?

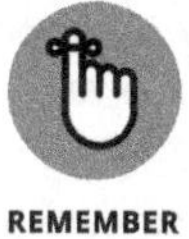

As long as you take excellent care of yourself and your partners, you can do whatever you want. Get grounded in what you want to do. Find some great possible candidates to share your lusts and longings with, create a fantastic consent container, and go for it.

Using Kink Fantasy Writing and Porn

Many people need more inputs or guideposts as they figure out their kinks. If your media consumption or social life has been highly controlled, you may have had little access to kink conversation, education, or social groups. Decades ago, kinksters had to exert a lot of effort to locate simple gateways to kink writing or media. Not today! You're fortunate to be conducting your kink investigation in an era when kink fantasy writing and porn are easily accessible.

Knowing where to access kink media

In Appendix B, you can find some of our favorite sources for your kink discovery process. But the best way to start is to just type keywords that describe your favorite kink fantasies into your search engine. You'll find many options that don't quite fit what you are looking for, and also a few gems that may lead you down a rabbit hole of additional searches.

Curate, curate, curate. When you find things that really align with your desires, keep digging. Depending on your interests, you may find it very easy to discover kink writing, storytellers, videos, and content creators whose work aligns with your fantasies.

This kind of discovery can give you many more creative ways to experience and consider your kink. It can help you find others who are in your kinky lane and kick off your process of building kink community.

Finding fan fiction and grassroots porn

So many sources of kink writing and visuals are commercial, which is fine. People who are talented get to make money and make their lives off of those talents. But fan fiction and grassroots (nonprofessional) porn sources that are free or nonmonetized are a blessing in kink spaces.

In these cases, people are mostly following their bliss, not the dollar. They are creating community and connection and digging deeply into their kinks to create joy among their peers. The Crash Pad Porn series comes to mind, where queer women created an ethical and egalitarian space to create their own porn. And then there's the Archive of Our Own, the largest nonprofit fan fiction site in the world, where you can find hundreds of thousands of kinky stories built around your favorite characters or celebrities — from Mr. Spock and Captain Kirk in Star Trek to Zelda and Link in the game, The Legend of Zelda— and tagged so you can easily find your favorite kinks.

Kink itself is outside of the box. Finding kink creators that offer their gifts outside of commercially-driven spaces can be incredibly enlivening.

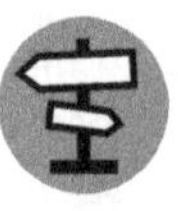

When I was in high school, I kept a semipublic diary on LiveJournal (an online blogging/diary platform and early example of social media.). One day, I published a list of my kinks, and my peers were like, "how do you even know?" And what they were really asking was, how could I pinpoint my interests without having engaged in real-life kink play? But I had read a lot of erotic fan fiction, and it led me to all manner of things I could feel turning me on. Some have faded. I'm no longer interested in cowboy costumes, for example. Maybe the most important discovery was what I found in Dragon Ball Z stories, in which Goku, the protagonist, and Vegeta, the bad boy, engaged in hurt/comfort, where they alternated between intense sex with angry words, spanking, and other forms of impact, and then moments of tender, loving cuddling. That's remained very high on my list of kinky likes. —**Jack**

Building on What You Know

If you are a true beginner in kink, you may be wondering where to start. Hopefully, the inventories and activities in this chapter (and elsewhere in the book) will give you a place to make internal reflections and begin to identify how you might enjoy and explore your kinky desires. But what then? How do you start to experiment or confirm that these wants are things that you actually want to play with?

As Jack notes in the previous story, you can *build on the known to discover the unknown.*

Moving between fantasy and real life

When should a kink fantasy just stay in your mind, and when is the right time to give a kink a try? Jack notes:

Two things about Jack's story are particularly useful here:

First, he found pals or people he liked but didn't necessarily have a romantic attachment to or partnership expectations. He was doing this with his high school theater buddies, but you can try it with friends who are also contemplating their kinks or one or more people you've met in a kink social group. Or you may consider trying things out with someone you've met through attending an educational class — say, a rope tying or play piercing demo.

Second, trying things out in a collective or experimental — rather than a 1-to-1 or emotionally high-stakes — environment can feel safer and comforting. Jack was in friendly cuddle piles in a van. Perhaps you could be at a kink social or at a kink resort or conference; maybe you're at a Leather bar and have found a hot kinkster, couple, or throuple who shares some of your kinky interests.

Think about how to make yourself comfortable and balance actual power — while perhaps trying to play with serious imbalances of power. Consider temperament, attraction, experience, and *je ne sais quoi* (French for *I don't know what*, for something special that's hard to define). You might be trying out different kinds of hurt or states of distress, but experimentation shouldn't be *actually* distressing or harmful.

Recognizing distress

When Jaime was growing up, she lived in a fairly high stress environment. Her mother had untreated depression and was often overwhelmed and would sometimes lash out. This was the '70s and corporal punishment was much more common. She received some of it; and her older brother got the very bad end of it, so she also observed a lot of hitting. Accordingly, Jaime spent a lot of her childhood in a high state of vigilance, which she notes:

personal relationships — if I sensed a threat, I would lash out verbally or physically. I became known as someone not to mess with.

All of this followed me into adulthood and into my adult kinky life where over time — thanks to many healing practitioners and beloved confidantes — I became aware of my state of distress. I could feel my pulse starting to quicken or the blood rushing in my ears. I could tell that something was off, when I wasn't feeling right. Instead of lashing out, I could start to ask myself questions about what was happening in the moment that was troubling me. I could walk myself back from my distress and figure out a next step. I could act instead of react.

Becoming aware that her activation was a distress response was a game-changer in Jaime's kink life and also her daily life. She could distinguish when something was safe and sexy from something that was veering toward harmful, or she wasn't capable of handling.

TIP

Recognizing the difference between sexy distress and actual harm is one of your superpowers in kink life. Being aware of how your history of distress lives in your body and recognizing what your internal alarm system is trying to communicate to you in kink scenarios — opens up your entire kink world.

Figuring out what's worth trying

Like all experimental projects, it's best to start with the easiest or most accessible thing. Maybe you're super turned on by elaborate scenes where you are in peril, like kidnappings. Consider an escalating series of kink experiments: perhaps start with a simple role-play where your play partner is a bit strict or edgy. Take in your emotional response. Discuss with your play partner afterward to figure out what worked best and what you'd like to build on.

If this works well for you, ramp up your experimentation to the next accessible "perilous" kink as you move toward your intense fantasy. In Chapter 8, you can find lots of ideas about how to create a simple consent container for fun experimentation.

Having a trusted confidante

It might be easier to try out kinks that you have fears about when you have at least one person who knows this about you. For example, Jaime loves being slapped. In the past, she had lengthy conversations with a childhood friend about being slapped when she was young. She wasn't sure she could stay present while being slapped, especially across the face. So Jaime talked through the possibilities with her friend before she could create satisfying and safe scene choreography with a play partner.

PLAY PARTNERS: OUR FAVORITE THINGS

What are good qualities in a play or scene partner? Here are a few of our favorites:

- **Great listener.** They're eager to hear about your kinks and your safety needs.

- **Grounded in their sexuality and their kinks.** This scene partner knows who they are.

- **Great sense of humor.** Let's have fun while we do all these intense things together!

- **Great communicator.** As you've described your wants and needs, this play partner is doing a great job introducing themselves. The exchange feels comfortable and it's relieving your anxiety as a novice to this kink.

While you're discovering what works for you, it's best to find people who already know you and your story. They know when you are lying to yourself or hiding. They can give you feedback you may not want to hear such as: *I don't think you are ready to try this yet.* They laugh with you about all of your dorkiness and silly worries, but never *at* you. Having a trusted friend to confide in means that you can recruit a scene partner who may not know you quite this well, or barely at all, because you have talked through all the possible outcomes with someone who treasures you.

If you don't have someone in mind at this time, don't worry! Chapter 11 has a great exercise on creating friendship and support pods.

Recognizing when you are over your line

When you are trying new things, sometimes it doesn't work out. What does this mean in the context of kink experiments? First and foremost, it means you know how to recognize and address when you have crossed into problematic or harmful territory, by knowing

>> You have a handle on yourself. You can track your own emotional and physical distress. (See the section, "Recognizing Distress" earlier in this chapter.)

>> You are capable of speaking up when you need to, even if you were so excited and sure this scenario would work — not matter if it disappoints a scene partner or disrupts an event.

MAKING A NEXT-LEVEL STRETCH

As a possessive Dom, there's a next level in terms of stretching myself that almost feels like too much to manage. So the times when I've done that, it's been rare — like inviting another masculine person into the mix with my partner(s).

That was something that was not my natural inclination. And so, I think communication, trust, a plan, and the belief that those all would be honored, and that there was space to talk about, around, and through it all.

There's a longevity arc that also made that possible; I did this with a long-term partner. That's not something I'm going to do with someone new. I can't just will myself through that.

And the other part of it is that I really am a community-person. So, if we do this, we're likely gonna cross paths at some point. And that's a secondary thing to manage because being who I am out in the work world or wherever, I'm a privacy lockdown kind of person. I think that also has impacted my arc, to be honest. **—M'Bwende**

Just because something doesn't work today doesn't mean it will never work. You can assess what happened or didn't happen with your scene partner and figure out what went wrong. You can stop, breathe, recoup, give yourself some time, and try again later — if that's what you want.

Dealing with fantasies that persist

Sometimes, after multiple failed tries, a kink fantasy may still feel compelling, even after realizing that it's not workable in person. Many kinksters experience this and may spend time grieving that while this fantasy is important and meaningful, it's not meant for real-time, interpersonal play.

This doesn't mean you can't still play with it. *Voyeurism* (see Appendix A) is an excellent alternative when you can't play with a treasured kink yourself. Creating a collection of favorite media depictions of your fantasy can be amazingly gratifying — giving yourself a library to enjoy. Solo fantasy time in your head is another option. Accepting where you are at emotionally and physically is a lifelong process for kinksters. Taking care of yourself in the kink scene means listening to yourself and getting creative about alternatives, even when you'd rather not.

Going where you've never been

One of the true joys of kink is finding yourself in new territories, over and over again. There's nothing quite like finding new kinks and new states of joy and intimacy over the stretch of your lifespan. If you've created a strong consent-building practice, found community and generative conversations about your kink, and developed some close friends and worthy play partners, you are in a good position to try new things and expand your kink repertoire.

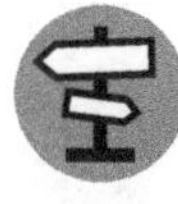

KINK
STORY

Top of the list in my fantasy wank bank is: gangbangs! So much about my desires and interests have changed over the years, but not gangbangs. I used to think this would be another fantasy for me to take to my grave, until I met a play partner who wanted to try it with me. We talked about all kinds of emotional and physical safety measures and showed up in a sex club to play. In many ways, the fantasy of a scene, especially one I had been crafting for years, is so much more elaborate and exciting than the real thing. But also, getting to actually experience it in the flesh was deeply gratifying and exhilarating. **—Aredvi**

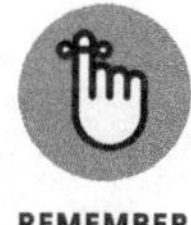

REMEMBER

The inventory you developed at the beginning of this chapter may have demonstrated that the desires you experience as pivotal to your sexuality today may shift over time. Your passions may change as you grow your capacity to identify, articulate, get support for, and share your kinks.

Chapter 6

Making Your Own Kink Meaning

Self-discovery in kinky life isn't linear or literal. Kink expression involves deep engagement with the unconscious, the hidden, and the suppressed. While outsiders often observe kinksters at play and wonder — what does it mean? Kinksters instead take the uncontainable, indescribable stuff of desire, fantasy, and taboo to create their own meaning.

In this chapter, we focus on the *what* and *how* of building your kinky life to help you find answers to important questions like: What do you want kink to bring into your life? How can you draw upon kink desire to help you build intimacy, hot sex, friendship, and/or family?

Delving into the complexities of these questions is how kinksters create meaningful kinky lives.

Mixing It Up: Attraction, Behavior, and Identity

In the mid '90s, Ritch Savin-Williams, Ph.D., noted that when researchers attempted to define or identify LGBTQ subjects, they often chose different avenues as their driving point for categorization. For example, sexologists looked at attraction (who people got hot for), health researchers looked at behavior (who people were actually having sex with), and feminists and cultural studies researchers looked at identity (how people described themselves and the communities these identities created around them).

Savin-Williams observed that none of these categorical frames overlaid precisely on the others. A research subject may be attracted to many genders, for example, while having sex with women and trans men, and yet identify as a lesbian. A man who describes himself as heterosexual may only seek women as romantic partners while frequently hooking up with men.

Savin-Williams noted that internalized *biphobia* (a fear and aversion toward being neither straight nor gay or of being sexual or making a life with many or any genders) drives some of these apparent contradictions. But in working with coaching clients, Jaime found another driver of this phenomenon: the prioritization of identify in the way people in the U.S. build their intimate lives. More than attraction and behavior, identity often drives how people move in the world — who they call their friends and loved ones and where they make their home. And this prioritizing of identity often masks a more complex life of attractions and sexual behavior.

Exploring the mixing bowl

A parallel phenomenon — crisscrossing or divergent streams of attraction, behavior, and identity — also operates in kink world. One kinkster may identify as a pain-seeking *switch* (someone who likes to both Top and bottom), for example, but plays mostly as a *submissive* or bottom. Yet while fantasizing, they are a ferocious, sadistic *Dominant* (Dom or Top).

Another kinkster identifies as a femme rope bunny, submitting to experienced masculine Rope Masters, while their fantasies are largely taken up with puppy play in which they are unbound, often rolling over and being told they are a "good boy." (See Chapter 4 for more information on pup and role-play.)

Yet another kinkster identifies as a strict Dom and is in great demand for their ability to induce subspace (see Chapter 10) for a wide variety of enthusiastic submissives. However, in out-of-town kink spaces where nobody knows them, they engage in age-play and identify as a baby.

Finally, a kinkster who strongly identifies a certain way is surprised to find themselves taking up new roles or practices adjacent to a kinkster they are attracted to and want to play with. For example, a Top who hates piss play is suddenly pissing all over the room.

So, what's going on in these situations? Here are just a few observations:

>> Similar to the biphobia observation by Savin-Williams, some kinksters are afraid of or repulsed by what they want and are hiding out in an identity descriptor that covers over their more complicated kink desires.

>> Other kinksters are repulsed by a particular fantasy (rather than concealing a phobia), which is *part of the kink*. They are keeping their desire private or underground because this actually amps up the intensity, making it even more kinky and satisfying.

>> Some kinksters are discovering or figuring themselves out, and this fantasy or hidden part of their kink practice may eventually move into in-person play.

>> Many kinksters are highly impacted by the desirability and desires of their partners, although we don't mean this in a codependent or "I will change to make you happy" kind of way. Instead, we mean it in a kinky, stretching, wonderful way, as in: "You are so hot! I can't believe my whole world of kink is shifting in this amazing moment." Therefore, their identities and desires shift as a result.

>> For kinksters who are exploring their genders or sexual orientations, kink fantasy or play in anonymous spaces may provide a first, safer arena for expressing or inhabiting their more authentic self.

>> And polar opposite to being phobic, kinksters may love this kinky part of themselves but only in their own private, solo play.

In all of the examples above, these kinksters are choosing the ways in which they relate to their kinks and the people they are intimate with.

Or, to stay with the mixing bowl analogy, the same kink ingredients can create very different kink meanings in different kinksters lives:

>> **Hiding.** Some kinksters will have a hard time coming to terms with what they want, over and over, throughout their lives. In this case, living double or triple lives will become part of who they are. (See also the next section, "The closet.")

>> **Reveling in repulsion.** Other kinksters may continue to put themselves in the path of an attraction/repulsion that it isn't actually an identity dilemma but a hot kink construction. This shapes who they are attracted to and what they pursue.

>> **Discovering.** Some kinksters will discover kinky desires or attractions that they didn't know about, often incorporating them into fantasy as a first step. Then, they'll find ways to integrate these new kinks into their practices, relationships, and identity.

>> **Shifting or building identity.** Drawing on the creativity and openness of kinky play, some kinksters will experiment with, develop, or express a buried sexuality or gender identity.

>> **Playing with multiplicity.** Other kinksters just love the whole circus. Their identities will shift with the winds; they might see themselves as "pan" or "omni" sexual and move through many practices, ways of being, and relationship forms throughout their lives.

>> **Keeping stuff for you.** Some kinksters revel in the private. They are not hiding or afraid. They are protective of the sacred space that gets them off like no other, meaning there are parts of themselves that no one sees.

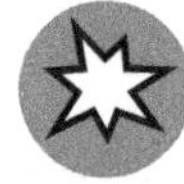

ACTIVITY

KEY INSIGHTS. In this exercise, take a moment to think about:

>> Whether the identities you share in public fully describe or work to conceal some of your kink attractions and practices.

>> Whether you're hiding or discovering or learning or shifting or preserving spaces for your kinks. How are/will you live out your kinky desires in the world?

>> What do your own discoveries so far say about *you*? What meanings are you making in your kink discovery process?

Be sure to document what you are learning about yourself, perhaps by writing down your insights in a journal, or making some art. You can also discuss what you are learning with a trusted friend.

The closet

It's difficult to live a life in the closet, and yet many of us do. Hiding your sexuality, family, race or ethnicity, genders, political positions, religion, and kinky practices from public view or behind a façade can become a way of life. Mostly, people hide to protect themselves and their loved ones or to keep their jobs or residences. Many people have been detained, displaced, or fired for revealing their true selves — in fact, Jaime has experienced this firsthand.

So, only you can assess when it's safe for you to openly live in a world that operates with multiple anti-sex, constraining, violent systems. Chapter 14 may help you consider whether to come out as kinky, but having even one confidante who really knows and understands you makes a tremendous difference if you are living a closeted kink life. It can turn the most dreadful loneliness into liberating privacy. Make it a point to try to find one.

Creating a Narrative

In this section, you can use the information you discovered about yourself in the previous Key Insights activity. If you are flipping through the book and haven't created a desire inventory yet, you may find it helpful to review the section, "Inventorying your intimate practices" in Chapter 5 to provide an even greater awareness of your desire narrative.

It's possible that your Key Insight activity yielded very little material at this point. Perhaps your have zero kink activities on your desire inventory. Maybe the only places you can find kink is around the edges of your fantasy life and arousal.

TIP

Kink fantasy and arousal is a fantastic starting place. Many kinksters live their entire kink lives in their brilliant minds, in their writing, or in their online or *parasocial relationships* (see Appendix A).The exercises that follow are designed to help you tell your story in a way that makes your life fuller, freer, and filled with people who love and understand you.

ACTIVITY

WHAT'S MY STORY? Reflect on your responses to the Key Insights activity in the previous section and your Chapter 5 desire inventory (if applicable) and answer the following questions:

>> If you were to tell a story based on all this information here, what's your two- or three-sentence summary?

>> What portrait would you create about yourself from these building blocks?

When Jaime thinks of her story, her response is: For more than 30 years, I have been an adventurous kinkster who has needed long stretches of solo time to integrate the knowledge I've gained from the revelatory experiences I've created with my kink partners. One big picture truth about me: when I can see that my partners are coming a bit unglued by my kinks, my instinct is to go harder.

My favorite thing has been discovering new parts of myself and my lovers through our kinks.

Jack's story is: I have been happiest when I have a few core anchor lovers, like a nesting partner and/or mainstay daddies, whom I trust to do intense kink play with full-body bondage. Additionally, I have always appreciated quantity over quality, trying new people and new ways to play at a quick clip; this includes people I meet through anonymously online or at in-person cruising spaces. I enjoy sampling kinks they like, even if they're not things I've necessarily been deeply drawn to in the past.

The next question is about meaning:

» What do your answers to the previous questions tell you about the impact kink has had on your life?

Jaime's answer: Kink intimacy has helped me heal, grow, and take more risks. Thanks to kink play, I'm not afraid of myself or my story anymore; I have a greater capacity for vulnerability in my intimate life. My mental health is much stronger! And outside the kink context, I'm better at saying no to things that don't work for me. I'm able to step into my full power as a partner in my family and at work.

While for Jack: Kink has helped me to continuously shed excess anxious energy that gets built up in my system. In periods of my life when I have had less access to play, my chronic worry and depression have been worse, and I've been less able to calm the whirring thoughts that get in the way of other aspects of my life. When I can hook up often and indulge my own and others' kinks, I wake up happier and more energized and I learn about the nooks and crannies of my desire that I might never have accessed otherwise.

The purpose of this question is to focus on *impact*. What is kink doing for you right now? Is it making your life better, fuller, and more pleasurable? If so, congratulations! Wherever you are on your kink path, you can build on that meaning.

However, if kink is only adding hardship to your story because you've chosen partners who are hard on you; if you're isolated, or if you're often in the presence of naysayers and judgmental authorities, seek community (see Chapter 13) or seek help (see Appendix B).

Finally, a closing question that leads into Activity 2: What might kink exploration make possible for you? Hmm? What do you think?

Everyone has stories they tell themselves. If you don't like yours, listen to yourself more deeply. Honor your insights. Tell yourself another.

FLIP THAT SCRIPT

Some years ago, Jaime had a Desire Mapping client who described herself as a *virgin* (see Appendix A) and reported that she had not had any satisfying intimate relationships. When we plotted her desire map, it was clear that she had dated a series of men who ignored what she wanted and acted as if she didn't know what she was doing sexually.

But when we dug deeper, it was clear that she *did know* what she wanted, which was control. As we discussed her fantasy life and how she created pleasure for herself, she preferred directing the sexual action. But when she was in-person with her dates, she felt like this desire was out of bounds. When she tried to articulate it, her partners shut her down.

Jaime directed her to dating platforms that draw a lot of kinksters, and where men who are interested in bossy or domineering women identify themselves and describe their wants. In just ten weeks of work together, my client created an entirely new narrative of her sexual story. At the close of our last session, she sent a drawing of herself standing on the top of the world in a superhero outfit, wielding a whip. The incapable virgin had been entirely displaced.

ACTIVITY

MY KINK FUTURE. The previous activity is an assessment of where you are now. This activity is aspirational, a projection into a hot kink future that you can imagine for yourself.

Here's how to do it:

1. **Find a quiet place to dream or imagine.** Minimize noise, interactions with people, and interruptions.

2. **Choose a best medium to create or record your imagined kink future.** Some people like to journal; others want to make art using markers, stickers, glitter, and other art supplies. Or perhaps you may want to voice-record a running narrative.

3. **Dream away!** Here are a few prompts to help you:

   - Who are you with in your kinky future? What are they like — their voice, features, most attractive qualities, or ways of speaking and interacting. What are their favorite kinky things? This could be a specific person or a kind of person. It could be your husband or the imaginary femme of your dreams.

- Where are you? What hot or dangerous or dreamy settings can you imagine for your kink utopia?

- What's your role? What's your place in the action when you are dreaming up the hottest kink connection you can imagine? What are your partners doing?

- What activities are you engaged in that you long for but have not yet tried?

- What are you doing *together*? Describe your favorite kink dynamic, sex positions, and/or romantic activities. In your wild kinky mind's eye, what's your pinnacle kink connection?

- How has pursing your kink desires effected your choice of partners, family structure and social life? Imagine the broader picture.

Tell yourself the story of your kinky future. Einstein said that the person with dreams is more powerful than the one with all the facts (and he was a guy who *loved* facts!). Envisioning your future self and relationships helps you to notice the spectacular nuances of pleasure that are already existing in your life.

Kink and Non-Monogamy or Polyamory

You may have noticed that when outlining many activities, there are references to your scene partners, or lovers, or playmates — usually plural. The kink discovery process often involves multiple people and relationships that may differ greatly from each other in terms of intimacy and commitment.

It's certainly not a must to be open to multiple lovers or play partners to be on a kink discovery path. Some of Jaime's clients do this quite happily and successfully within a monogamous relationship that does not involve others in any way. Others even incorporate the sexual and intimate exclusivity of their relationship into their kink play. Two people can be inventive scene partners and spouses for life, if that's your preferred relationship form.

However, having multiple teachers, experimental playmates, and lovers is a very common practice in the kink world. And if you want to learn more about polyamory, you can pick up Jaime's book, *Polyamory For Dummies*.

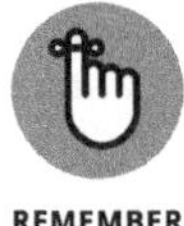

You know best how to forge your own kink discovery path. You can do that solo — entirely on your own — or with one trustworthy partner or many people with whom you share various kinds of intimacy and kinky play. It's your call.

Discovering That There Is No Normal

A relief that many kinksters come to is that there is no "normal" or customary in kink sexuality. On any given day, asking a search engine to list the top 20 kinks results in an ever-evolving list of practices that are being tried out all across the world.

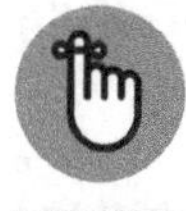

Despite the condemning, pointed fingers of various social and religious authorities, kink persists and evolves.

Appreciating kink evolutions

Kinky people all over the world explore and find each other. Unheralded kinky practices are revealed to the broader community, get adopted by others, and become popular. In the next week or month or year, something else surfaces and the whole process begins again. One year it's a love of *MILFs* (Mom or Mommy I Would Love to F*ck) and the next it's *breath play* (see Appendix A).

In a world of escalating insecurity and shrinking opportunity, endless and ever-changing versions of kink create a place of hope and expansive possibility for many kinksters.

KINK CURIOSITIES. In this activity, you can go to the search engine or conversational community of your choice and plug in your top three kink curiosities. One kinkster's list might look like this:

>> Is cosplay a kink?

>> What are the top ten kinks in the U.S. (or in the country you reside in)?

>> Do people fetishize or obsess over certain sensations? Like what?

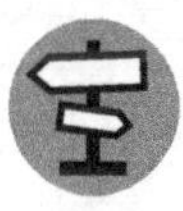

I remember the first time I realized that just because you're disgusted by something doesn't mean you're not into it. Actually, I still get pretty disgusted when people spit in my mouth. I'm ill! Like, *why are you doing that?* Because growing up, you weren't supposed to spit. Spitting is one of the worst things you can do to someone.

So when it happened, I realized the things that you think might disgust you or might be triggering to you can also be very pleasurable. When I've allowed my nervous system to move beyond that frozen place from the initial experience of disgust, it feels like my kink play is a kind of completion. **—Romeo**

Playing with taboos is hot

Why are taboos so compelling? Despite all prohibitions against enacting them, why do kinksters constantly cross the lines that society has drawn?

The most formal, shy kinkster you've ever meet will report that they love incest play. The kindest, sweetest of them all will be a killer with a whip in hand. A kinkster who lives in a religious order will have the filthiest and most degrading mouth you've ever imagined when addressing their subs in a scene.

There's nothing that brings a kinkster more pleasure than obliterating the lines that others have drawn for you about what's acceptable, or what you can and cannot have. Kink is all about breaking out and rejecting boundaries, especially around authority and conformity. So don't be surprised when you see it. As long as your taboo-breaking causes no one harm, it really doesn't matter what anyone else thinks about it.

Meaning Happens in Relationship

While you may decide that solo kinky life is for you (and if so, *Bravo!*), the vast majority of kinksters live their kink lives in relationships with others. Even solo kink practitioners may have a thriving set of intimates who discuss and share info on their kinks. Supportive, mutually enlivening relationships are a great blessing in kink life because so much meaning happens in unpredictable intimate exchanges (see more on this in Chapters 10 and 13).

Sharing your inner yearnings, revealing yourself to someone you trust and/or love involves vulnerability, which is the currency of kink. Some would say that kink life chases and cherishes vulnerability above all else. Kinksters are nothing if not the ultimate seekers of the banished and the unknown, those places where vulnerability lives.

There are so many ways to meaningfully share yourself in kink life, such as:

>> Reveal and discuss your discoveries with friends or confidantes.

>> Tell a potential play partner about your attraction to them or your burning kink desire.

>> Ask for support from a helping professional, a social group, or an intimate friend to figure out how to play with your kinks.

>> Ask to try things out with a potential scene partner, lover, of kinky friend.

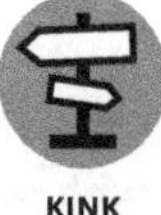

My favorite kink wing person is a gay man, a Dom who I just tell everything. As a Midwestern "straight" woman with seriously twisted desires, I've had a hard time finding friends who could listen to all the things I want to explore. But because he's coming at kink from a different gender and sexual orientation and even family structure — he is polyamorous and so far, I'm monogamous — it's just freed me up to tell the truth. He has no agendas around my kinky fantasies. He's delighted by them! It's like being on a study abroad program. *In my country, we do X, but I'm so glad to be here in your country where I can stretch and learn a new language and maybe try doing Y.* —**Anonymous**

Finding Meaning Through Research

Another way to find meaning in your kink expression is to place yourself in the larger story of kink history and practice. Far from being a fad or trend, kinky ways of being have been recorded for hundreds, and even thousands of years. If you want to learn more about famous kinksters across millennia, go to Chapter 18.

If you are experiencing your kink solo or feel like it separates you from others, understanding kink history can break you out of isolation and help you see your desires and practices in the larger context of human sexual expression.

In this next section, you can survey the work of prominent sexologists to note how scholarly thinking and research on kink has evolved over time.

Moving from von Krafft-Ebing to Kinsey to Foucault

Trailblazing sexologists and philosophers have thought a lot about kink over the past 200 years, illuminating an astonishing range of kink practices. In the mid-1880s, Richard von Krafft-Ebing began to articulate a perspective on "deviant" sexuality that moved away from characterizing kink as a mental disorder and more toward a variation of human sexuality. He interviewed thousands of research subjects as a professor at the universities of Graz (1872–89) and Vienna (1889–1902) and was considered one of the most prominent psychiatrists in Central Europe.

Nearly a century later in the U.S., Alfred Kinsey's research in the 1940s and '50s built on the work of Krafft-Ebing. Kinsey and his team gained fame for the sheer volume of their subjects and for shattering myths, including their finding that sex outside of marriage was common.

Interpreting the work of the masters

In the '70s, famed French philosopher Michel Foucault noted that Krafft-Ebing and Kinsey's research amplified a kind of medicalized obsession with sexuality, which established avenues of medical surveillance and control. Foucault demonstrated that sexology research has often been used to criminalize and constrain different people and sexual practices, rather than create more space for exploration or acceptance.

Nonetheless, one of the great values in Kraft Ebing's and Kinsey's work in particular, was the creation and respect for individual stories or case studies, which described thousands upon thousands of different sexual practices and desires, thereby creating a massive archive of what we refer to today as a kink.

While Krafft-Ebing set out to record "sexual perversions," the vastness of his and Kinsey's work countered the idea of perversion by presenting seemingly unending variations — a vibrant canvas of sexual diversity. Krafft-Ebing's and Kinsey's research has been drawn on by contemporary scholars to rethink what even constitutes "normal" sex and how sex and desire function to create meaning in human social, intimate, and family life.

TIP

If you are feeling like you're the only one with a particular kink, check out the history of sexuality. Look into various interpretations of numerous kink practices throughout time as well as many kinksters' impact on social and sexual history (see Chapter 18).

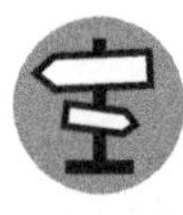

KINK STORY

As a young feminist, I struggled with my interest in kink. I was ashamed of being turned on by patriarchal behavior. One day a friend of mine handed me some articles that looked at the history of kink, and I started to understand it as more historically rooted than I had imagined. I began investigating the indigenous history of kinky practices — both in Iran, where I grew up, and within the Americas. I quickly learned that playing with pain, pleasure, bondage, impact, and other forms of intense and creative practices is nothing new, modern, or Western. It was truly liberating to see that kink can be yet another way for me to tap into ancestral wisdom. **—Aredvi**

Kink archives

Kink archives perform the crucial work of documenting the existence and persistence of BDSM, Leather, fetish and kink communities (see Chapter 4 for more on these communities). Places like the Leather Museum and Archives in Chicago and The Bishop Gate's Institute in the UK have collected significant kink archives of community organizations, personal photos, and play spaces. These attest to the explosion of kink culture and organizing from the 1970s to the present, but also catalogue kink relationships that date as far back as the mid-1800s. The archives are a powerful testament to the seemingly endless forms kink has taken on over centuries, and the likelihood that kink practices are as old as humanity itself.

KINK STORY

WRITING THE KINK PRESENT

In my life, finding kink connections among writers, activists, and artists that I admire has made me braver and more celebratory about my kinks. Since I came of age in the 1980s, early pro-sex classics like Sheree Hite's *Hite Report* were very important to me because they broke through mythologies about acceptable women's sexuality. More recently, adrienne maree brown's *Pleasure Activism* helped me see my kink in the context of fighting back against authoritarians; Miranda July's *All Fours* affirmed my experience in my late 40s, when my kinky libido was off the charts. Substacks from people like Susie Bright whose sex activism has carved out a path for a generation of sex activists make me realize there's no endpoint to growing — personally or politically — in sexual liberation. And Audre Lorde's landmark essay in the '70s, *The Erotic Is Power* still guides so much sex and racial justice activism around the globe. **—Jaime**

Chapter 7

Honing Your Communication Skills

When we think about what will really serve you as a kink communicator, self-knowledge and self-advocacy — or knowing what you need and how to ask for it — are the two key components of success.

Accordingly, understanding communication styles and developing awareness of your specific obstacles, such as speaking up, and staying present will be game-changers for you in your kink conversations and relationships.

In this chapter, you can explore two crucial facets of kink communication: The first is your communication style, and the second is your formative history of attachment in pivotal relationships. With this knowledge, you can look closely at your communication strengths and roadblocks, and work to improve your skills.

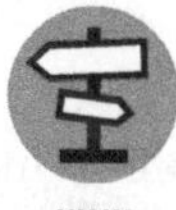

KINK
STORY

Communicating about kink is not as easy as some might think. Many people assume that if you're liberated enough to explore kinks, you can probably talk openly about all things sex-related. This, sadly, is not true. When done openly and with intention, communicating about kink can be a beautiful, magical experience that opens pathways for all kinds of exploration, even outside of kink. However, when approached poorly — from a place of fear or dishonesty — it can cause havoc, harm relationships, end the best of friendships, and demolish kinky possibilities. **—Rox**

In kink life, there are a lot of emotionally sensitive moments, whether in an intensely vulnerable kink scene or at a coffee date, co-creating the terms of a future sexy engagement. You owe it to yourself and your partners to dig into your story and improve your communication skills. Your kink relationships will always be the better for it.

Identifying Your Personality Traits

How would you describe yourself as a communicator? What kind of support do you need to communicate well and enjoy your kinky life? The following sections help you think about the different ways you tend to operate, so you can increase your self-awareness about your personality traits and their impact on your ways of communicating.

Being an introvert versus an extrovert

An important thing to note in terms of communication styles is the introvert/extrovert mix in your partnerships or kink connections. Introverts and extroverts approach social and intimate interactions differently, and they also need different kinds of support to stay present and enjoy themselves. Appreciating rather than denying or judging these differences is a strong step toward connecting with your partners.

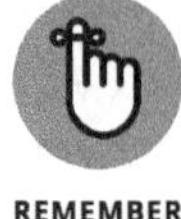

The simplest way to identify an introvert or extrovert is not to assess how you operate at a party — some introverts are wildly chatty among the people they love best, for example — but rather how you refuel and recoup. Consider the following:

>> **Introverts.** People who thrive and revive on alone time and the power to define their space. Introverts tend to need a *lot* of space and time alone to take in sensitive information, process its meaning, and respond.

>> **Extroverts.** People who thrive and revive on feedback, engagement, and the energy of others. Extroverts tend to solve problems out loud, in-the-moment, through active conversation and engagement.

Taking alone-time to reflect upon a high-conflict relationship problem makes no sense at all to an extrovert, whereas it may feel like the only way to survive for an introvert.

THE MYERS-BRIGGS ASSESSMENT AND THE WORKPLACE

Mother-daughter team Katherine Cook Briggs and Isabel Myers created the world's most popular sorter of introverts and extroverts in the 1950s, known as the *Myers-Briggs Type Indicator* (MBTI).

These two trained psychologists were motivated by Myers's experience in World War II, where she often saw the impacts of mismatched personality types on teams that were charged with extremely sensitive war projects. Together, Myers and Briggs hoped to shine a light on the very different ways that workers experience each other and the tasks at hand. They also aimed to shift analyses of the personality spectrum that often pit one communication type against each other, as in: extroverts, good; introverts, bad.

A lot of workplaces have come to understand the power of using the MBTI to identify styles of engagement to improve the productivity of their teams. Jaime remembers one work retreat when introverts were encouraged to say everything they'd ever wanted to say to the extroverts and vice versa. For example, they said something like this:

- **Introverts:** "Stop acting like I have no social skills. I'm choosing not to talk — I'm not a child."

- **Extroverts:** "Appreciate me for my engaging conversational skills at all of these demanding public events. And stop acting like I'm ruining your day when I'm just happy to talk to you."

The airing of these grievances surprised everyone on both sides of the introvert/extrovert spectrum. Who knew that work colleagues were carrying such resentments? The session helped the group recalibrate and understand the ways that everyone had been hard on other colleagues. Jaime found this exercise to be very useful in her practice as she watched introverts and extroverts struggle with each other in a kink dynamic or relationship.

Eyeing the MBTI and how you can use it

Today, managers use the MBTI results to determine the introvert/extrovert mix in their teams as well as other traits such as sensing/intuiting, feeling/thinking, and judging/perceiving.

If you've taken the MBTI, you may already have a sense of your profile and its possible meanings for you as a kink communicator. If you haven't taken the assessment or need a refresher, Figure 7-1 explains the 16 different MBTI personality types, which can give you a snapshot of who you are and how you move in the world.

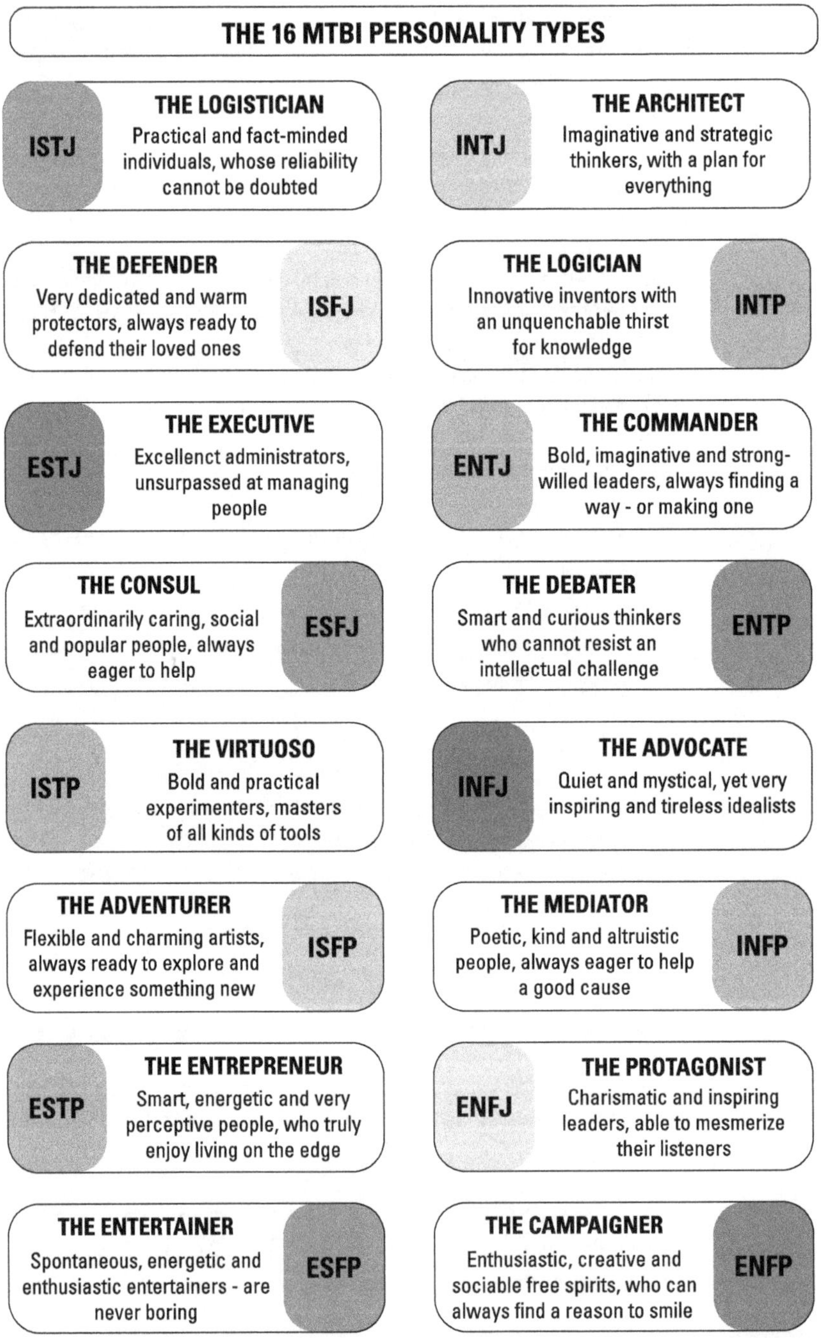

FIGURE 7-1: The 16 MBTI types.

badproject/Adobe Stock Photos

For years, experts suggested that MBTI results were a definitive and unchanging evaluation of character, but then people who took the assessment over time saw their results shift as they aged. In Jaime's case, she found that when she took the assessment at work, she scored differently from when she took it in relationship contexts. She is an ENTP (the Debater) or ENTJ (the Commander) at work and an INFP (the Mediator) or ENFP (the Campaigner) in her personal life. This made so much sense — the parts of Jaime's personality that take over at work and at home are suited to the tasks at hand. Communicating in intimate or familial situations brings very different strengths to life.

If you suspect that your persona or engagement strategies change between your work and home life, answer the MBTI questions by thinking about how you operate in your social life rather than how you solve problems at work (You can find more information about the MBTI at www.mbtionline.com).

Share and compare your assessments with your potential kink partners. Your MBTI may give you insights into communication issues that recur or seem to be in the way of creating the kinky scenes you want.

Communicating while neurodivergent

Over the past ten years, people who identify as neurodivergent have become more visible in the U.S., through sharing their stories about how they experience the world. Being *neurodivergent* (or neuro*atypical*) relates to a spectrum of experience where a person's brain processes information differently from other (neuro*typical*) people. The category includes but isn't limited to people with autism, attention deficit and hyperactivity (ADHD), giftedness, and so on.

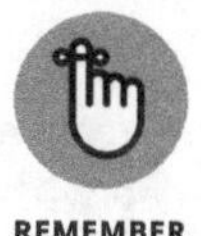

It's very likely that you'll run into neurodivergent communicators as you look for kinky lovers and play partners. While the theories about *why* are endless, the focus should be on *what* a neurodivergent person may need or do in different situations.

For example, people who have ADHD often process information by jumping from one sensory input to another; they can have difficulty sitting still or staying with a single thread of conversation. Some people may rarely complete their tasks or show up to work on time. Other neurodivergent partners may have limited verbal communication skills or — at another end of the spectrum — demonstrate tremendous verbal capacity.

Figure 7-2 on autism, ADHD, and giftedness, adapted from the work of Katy Higgins Lee, MTF, describes many common, overlapping experiences of neurodivergent individuals. As you can see, there are many sensory, emotional, and behavioral experiences here that can come into play when communicating.

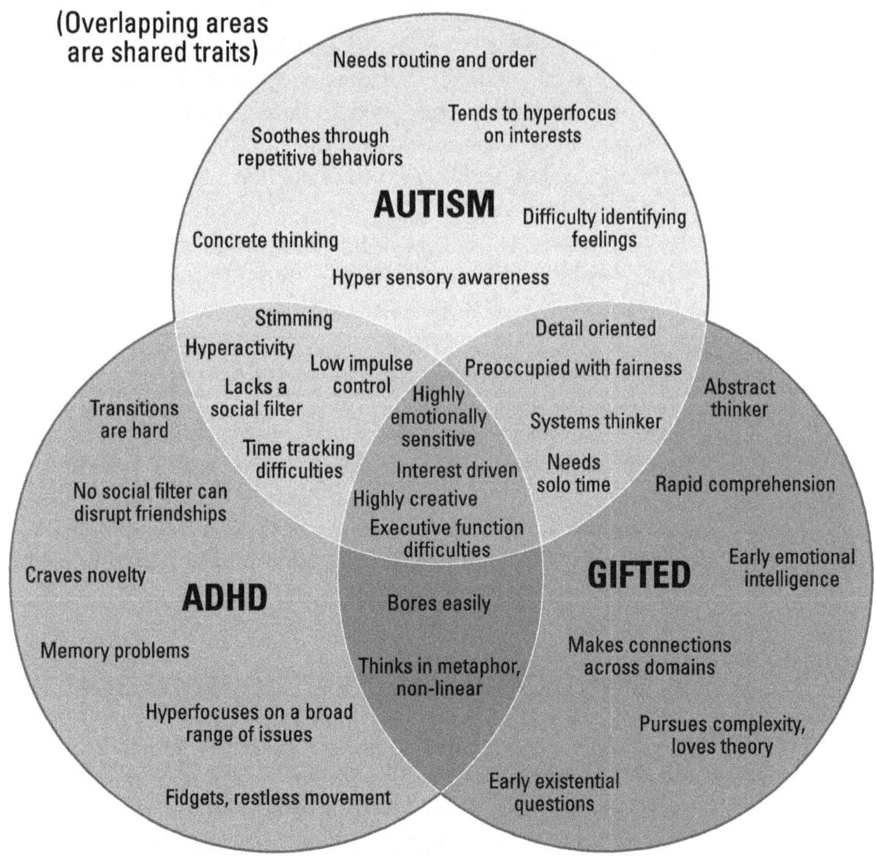

FIGURE 7-2:
Autism, ADHD, Giftedness Venn diagram.

Kathryn H. Lee / https://www.katyhigginslee.com/giftedness-autism-adhdvenn-diagram-pdf-free-download / Last accessed on Sep 09, 2025

TIP

If you or a kink partner identifies as neurodivergent, the best course of action is to create a space together to share how your or their specific neurodivergent traits impact intimacy and connection. Then, you can decide what's needed within your communication practices so that everyone feels heard and supported. In the absence of this kind of sharing, you're setting yourself up for communication miscues and blunders.

A neurotypical partner, for example, may interpret an autistic partner's lack of eye contact during a scene as disconnect or distress. Or a neurotypical partner may receive a neurodivergent partner's discussion about a particular kink, which includes lengthy description and a cascading series of facts, as nervousness or a problem.

REMEMBER

You don't know what you don't know. Making assumptions about the meanings behind a partner's communication practices is never a better course of action than hearing directly from them about their experiences.

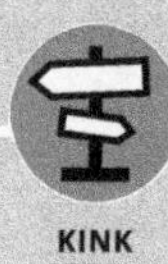

I WAS SO FOCUSED ON THE DETAILS; I MISSED THAT I WASN'T OKAY

Once I was in the middle of a rope scene I had really, really wanted to orchestrate and things unexpectedly shifted for me. The first sign that I was not okay was that I had stopped talking during the scene and became very focused on minute details of how I was tying the ropes — how it all looked and sat on my submissive's (sub's) body, wanting it all to look "perfect." Every time I looked at my work and noticed that it was not perfect, I became more and more frustrated and physically reactive. My heart started to race, I started to panic, and it took me a while to even realize that my scene partner was asking me if I was okay. What eventually snapped me out of it was the person sitting up and kind of shaking me and asking if we needed to stop and I told them yes.

I'm really grateful that this human wanted to talk about it all afterwards because I surely did not. I felt pretty embarrassed but eventually was able to communicate that I had been putting a lot of pressure on myself for the scene to look like this fantasy I had in my head, and when it didn't, I became activated and panicked. To this day, I can still hear the way they laughed and said "wouldn't it be great if everything in our heads were actually the same in real life." —**Bishop**

If a partner's communication style seems disconnected or at odds with yours, speak up. Investigate. Your best results as a communicator come when you put yourself in a position to share, learn, and grow.

Looking at Your Communication Style

If you grew up in a family or caregiver situation with a lot of yelling and arguing, or if there was constant tension — where you felt like you had to change your behavior all the time to prevent a blowup — you've likely developed a set of coping skills that you aren't even aware of. In this section, you can look more closely at how the set of skills you grew as a child is supporting or hampering your kink communication.

Responding to childhood trauma

Over the years, Jaime has grown a lot of respect for her childhood coping skills. She was raised in a household where her parents hid most of their problems, and then occasionally, they couldn't contain their conflicts, and her mother would yell at everyone while her dad made a hasty exit. Additionally, like many people of their generation, Jaime's parents believed in *corporal punishment* (see Appendix A).

So, when it came time to figure out how all of this impacted her present-day relationships, theories about childhood trauma and communication helped. (Chapter 11 discusses trauma survivors and kink in greater detail.)

Theorists like Judith Hermann and Gabor Maté have outlined the four basic responses of adults who had to navigate emotionally fraught or physically abusive childhood households, and they are *fight, flight, freeze,* or *fawn.*

Finding out which mode of communication (or noncommunication) you slip into when conflict arises is important because your childhood experiences can influence the way you communicate today. Check out the following responses:

>> **Fight:** When the going gets tough, you come back verbally swinging. Your partners say they never win an argument with you. Once activated, you're going to defend yourself to your last breath.

>> **Flight:** As the voices rise in the room, you slowly disappear. By the time conflict is high, you've probably got your hat and coat on and are out the door.

>> **Freeze:** As the argument unfolds, you're here but not here. Maybe you're on the ceiling when your partner gets agitated or starts to raise their voice. What's being said? Who knows. You're frozen.

>> **Fawn:** You may tell jokes when emotions start to heat up, trying to distract your partner from their pain, or tamping down their fury. Or maybe you're telling a fellow kinkster that you are in conflict with how wonderful they are and that everything is going to be okay because everything is fine . . . just fine.

Not being able to communicate in the moment when emotions run high or when trust has been breached is okay. You can take a break and figure out what you need to reset. You can seek support. However, sabotaging or abandoning a kink collaborative process altogether isn't okay.

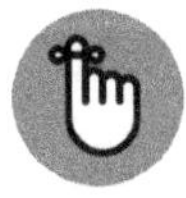

Being a good communicator means knowing how to inform your partner(s) about what's happening in your body, brain, and heart. Then, you can eventually move away from a traumatic activation prompted by the past, so that you can face whatever your needs are in the present.

Discovering the ways you communicate

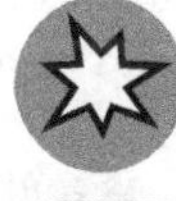

ACTIVITY

When you're ready to discover how your childhood story is impacting your present-day communication, ask yourself the following questions about how you communicate:

» On a scale of 1 to 5, with 5 being very often, how often did you experience conflict in your family of origin or childhood household?

» How was conflict resolved?

» How did you react to conflict in your family? What was your role during family arguments or violence?

» Did anyone else take care of you when you were scared or upset? How?

» How did you take care of yourself when you were scared or upset?

» When you reflect on these answers, do you see yourself as a person who fights, flees, freezes, or fawns (as described in the previous section)?

This exercise provides some insight that will be a lot to take in. Breathe. Consider how you may best tackle this exercise. By yourself? With a partner? Maybe you need a trained professional to help sort through these questions. Looking at how old hurts are still driving how you operate today with people you love may be difficult.

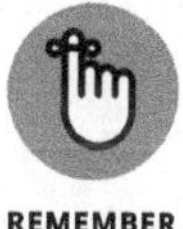

REMEMBER

It's so important in kink communication to know how your past is impacting your present so you can set boundaries, build a strong consent container (see Chapter 8), and enjoy a scene as it unfolds.

The good news is that your communication style or difficulties with reactivity aren't set in stone. As long as you're open to the truth of your story, seek support to heal and make changes, and then take responsibility for yourself and the impact of your behavior — you can improve as a communicator. You can step up to your kink desires with confidence.

Dealing with mental health challenges

For many people, their ancestors and parents survived poverty, violence, and displacement, which has had a significant impact on mental health over generations. Recent advances in the field of *epigenetics* demonstrate that intergenerational trauma and mental illness have an impact on genetic expression.

And that doesn't even account for people's day-to-day experiences.

Many of us are direct survivors of multiple systems of violence, which has had a massive impact on our mental health. The mental health advocacy organization National Alliance on Mental Illness (NAMI) estimates that 20 percent or one in five people in the United States experience some kind of mental illness every year.

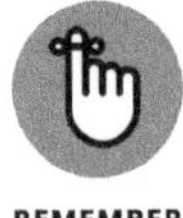

If you're part of that 20 percent, the important thing to remember is that people with significant mental illness pursue kink connections of all kinds, every day, just like everyone else.

Some mental illnesses present particular hardships around kink relationships — people suffering from *dissociative disorders* (see Chapter 10 for more on dissociation) and addictions have a difficult time showing up and being consistent. This can have a big impact on consent conversations in the lead-up to a kink engagement, or as your needs unfold in a kink scene. People with complex *post-traumatic stress disorder* (PTSD; present-day experiences activate an emotional or embodied response to traumatic events in the past) struggle with unpredictable reactions when they're intimate or vulnerable. If your kink scenes knock into unaddressed trauma, your partner might experience tremendous distress. (See Chapter 11 for more information on trauma survivors).

If you or your play partner has a significant mental illness, you will want to take extra care in creating your consent container and plans for unpredictable responses and distress while in a scene.

But nothing thrills your wronged and deprived ancestors like your healing and success. Check out the pod mapping discussion in Chapter 11 to think about and how to build the support you need. And go get that kinky life!

Applying Attachment Theory to Kink Play

Similar to applying a fight-or-flight lens to your communication style, discussed earlier in this chapter, investigating your formative attachment story can provide clues about your challenges as you build intimacy and trust in kink relationships. The following sections explore attachment theory and consider how it may apply to you.

Defining attachment theory

Research suggests that what happened between infancy up to age 5 has a significant impact on a person's ability to trust and attach as an adult. *Attachment theory* investigates the connection between your formative attachments — those with your parents and other close caregivers — and your patterns in relating intimately as an adult.

BOWLBY AND AINSWORTH'S ATTACHMENT THEORY

In 1958, psychologists John Bowlby and Mary Ainsworth developed a theory of attachment based in part on experiments wherein a mother and infant established a play space in an observational setting, and then the mother exited the room. Researchers monitored escalating anxiety in the child, and the mother returned to offer comfort. This test established the psychological term *separation anxiety* and created categories of attachment based on the baby's connection to the mother and its ability to reestablish a secure bond. (These terms are described in greater detail later in this chapter.)

While becoming one of the most highly referenced works on attachment and mental health in children and adults in the world, Bowlby's and Ainsworth's work had significant flaws. Their ideas about attachment hinge on the mother as the sole caregiver, much like other mid-century studies, to suggest that a mother's relationship to a child is singular and all-determining. The experiment fails to consider that a child may have more than one significant caregiver of any gender and also doesn't consider what kind of systemic stresses might impact a child-caregiver bond, such as poverty, violence, displacement, and so on. Bowlby and Ainsworth's work is aimed at one mother's success at connection or empathy in an isolated situation.

(continued)

(continued)

Despite these limitations, this research opened a pathway to considering the effects of disruptive attachment on children as they move through crucial early stages of development. Accordingly, as you look at the attachment categories that we introduce later in this chapter, you can think about your attachment story in terms of your closest caregivers through your formative years, but also at whether your family were targets of institutional violence, discrimination, and/or poverty. All of these factors come together to influence your attachment story.

Investigating early childhood attachment

In this section, you can undertake an exercise to help uncover your attachment story. By sifting through your history to understand your present-day challenges, you may discover ways that your unconscious burdens are getting in the way of navigating intimacy.

ACTIVITY

MY ATTACHMENT STORY. Use a dedicated journal for this exercise. Find a private space and be sure to give yourself time to answer the following questions because they may bring up memories you haven't visited for a long while.

» What do you know about your early attachment story? Can you ask a parent or caregiver about the circumstances surrounding your early childhood? Write down what you know about the environment. Here are some specific questions to consider:

- Was your birth uneventful? Were you able to be with your parents or separated from them at the start of your life?

- Did your family have enough resources to care for you?

- Was anyone in your household very sick or in a crisis when you were young?

- Were people in the family targeted by police or the government?

- Was your family ever displaced from their housing?

- Was there violence in your home? Were any of your parents harmed?

- Were you harmed?

» When you think about your earliest memories as a baby, toddler, or preschooler, what is the emotional content of these memories?

- Are you laughing?

- Are you crying?

- Are you frightened?

- Are you wrapped in the arms of someone who loves you?

- Who in your earliest memories created a place of comfort?

» When you think about times that you were scared or hurt as a very young child, who is there for you?

- What happened in this memory?

- Who intervened?

- What was your connection like?

- Do you remember being comforted?

- How would you describe the resolution of this hurtful experience?

You can bookend this activity with a phone call or text a dear friend, if you need emotional support afterward.

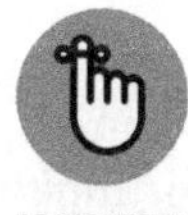

REMEMBER

Investigations like this can be multilayered and take some time. You may have to revisit these questions again and again. Just allow yourself to move through your memories and know what you know. You may want to get information from siblings and family members to round out your inquiry.

Take all these clues and keep them together. Having this information handy can be helpful as you look through the attachment categories discussed later in the section "Looking Closer at Attachment Styles."

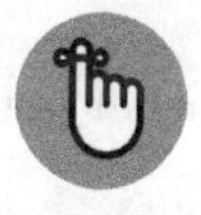

REMEMBER

Discovering your attachment story might be difficult, but denying your attachment wounds cripples your ability to attach.

Pretending that you don't have attachment wounds won't make them go away and in fact will make addressing attachment challenges more difficult as you deny and deflect your attachment barriers with your partners.

Kink relationships can surface attachment wounds because kinksters are often playing in or near the territories where these wounds were established. If your father left your family when you were a child, for example, and you have a Daddy kink, your kink yearnings to play with attention, discipline, and abandonment with your kink Daddy may open the door to feelings of hurt or abandonment you were not able to fully process as a young person. Or if you've survived a miscarriage and you have a pregnancy kink and play at being impregnated — this kind of play may reveal unexplored grief. The beauty of kink play is that it often reveals your hidden complex inner life to you.

Learning more about your attachment story can create deeper and more meaning-ful play in your kink life.

The challenge of kink play is that you need to find caring partners who can attend to the possible activation of your attachment wounds and take great care of you. Additionally, you need to be resourceful yourself, through recognizing when these kind of vulnerable openings occur and being able to signal to a partner what you need.

Integrating your attachment story

As you gain important insight about your attachment story, the next step is integrating the information and taking care of yourself. Many people have been discouraged from thinking too deeply about their attachment stories by parents and caregivers. You may have been told, "the past is in the past." Some of this misdirection may have been the result of a misguided protectiveness. In previous generations, a lot of parents were advised to hide hard truths from their children.

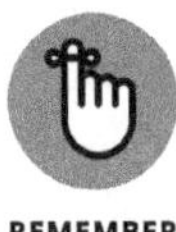

Investigating your attachment story can be difficult. Many of Jaime's clients have parents who have lied or withheld significant information thinking that they were shielding their children. But these truths live in your body and psyche. Regardless of whether your parents reveal the honest narrative of your early childhood, experiences of early attachment and disconnect persist in your adult capacity to connect, be intimate, and sustain your close friendships and partnerships.

Going back to your childhood and finding the truth of your experience is okay, even if nobody in your family wants you to do this.

The following is Jaime's attachment story:

> When my mother died, I went into a deep depression and had to seek psychiatric help. One of the first questions that my psychiatrist had for me was about the environment I experienced as a child. My mother had been an alternately very loving and volatile presence in my childhood, and I didn't see what help it would be to ask my dad for more information about this. He was grieving the loss of a partner of nearly 40 years, and I was sure I had all the necessary pieces of the story. Nonetheless, my psychiatrist insisted that I call him. When we finally connected, my dad explained that my mother had been a survivor of major depression (news to me) and had been hospitalized against her will after my brother's birth in the late 1950s. The doctors had forced my mom to undergo electroconvulsive therapy, which at the time was a much more brutal treatment than it is today.

This information was devastating, but it also explained a lot. I asked if my mom took medication after her hospitalization, and he said, "No, the depression never came back." In just this short phone call, my mother's lifelong rigidity and harshness as a parent came into an entirely new light. She hadn't been arbitrary or mean with me, she had been scared witless, so much so that she let everyone around her believe she didn't need any further treatment.

Getting this part of my attachment story helped me do two important things:

- Reevaluate my mother as a person in an isolating, heroic struggle to stay out of the hospital and stay with us. She wasn't being callous or dismissive; she was sick and struggling fiercely to function so that nobody would notice her pain or force her to go back to treatment.

- Reevaluate myself as a child who had a compromised primary caregiver. My attachment environment was full of anxiety, fear, loneliness, and anger. A lot of the struggles in my adult intimate attachments suddenly made sense. This one piece of information cemented my commitment to getting a therapist who understood the impact of parental mental illness on a child.

- Reorient myself to my deep need for attention in my kinky play. Getting more of my formative story helped me understand that I'd hidden a lot of my childhood feelings of terror and abandonment. Knowing this, I began to craft kinky scenarios with my partners that touched on this wound, but also took fantastic care of me. My kinky practices became more meaningful in the aftermath of finding this part of my attachment story.

ATTACHMENT INVESTIGATION. Here are a few questions that can help you dig deeper into your attachment story:

>> Ask your parent, caregiver, siblings, or even an aunt or uncle about attachment disruptions that you remember. Ask them if they remember what happened. Try to uncover new details from others' perspectives in the family.

>> Ask if the family member recalls how you responded to this disruption. Again, get any details you can gather. This person's memories may not be entirely accurate, but they're recollections based in your family system and can give you important perspective.

>> Make a list of three new insights you've gained about your attachment story by asking for others' perceptions of your story. They can be helpful clues as you figure out your attachment style.

Looking Closer at Attachment Styles

In this section, you can look through some established categories on attachment to help identify where you may sit on the attachment spectrum. These classifications can give you some insight about common challenges that arise from your attachment type. From there, you can consider what kind of support you may need to build the kind of closeness and intimacy you want.

Identifying the attachment styles

Researchers have observed family relationships and attachment styles over the years and have developed four core categories. The following list delves into each one:

>> **Secure attachment.** If you have a secure attachment style, you likely had very abundant and consistent caregiving when you were young. Your family's economic and social situation was likely stable and supported. When you reached out for comfort, your parent or caregivers often affirmed your experience and held you close until you felt better.

> As adults, secure attachers tend to be comfortable with intimacy and have confidence in their relationships. They find it relatively easy to be vulnerable and take risks. And although breakups may be painful, as they are for all people, secure attachers are less likely to beat themselves up or to fall into deep, prolonged regret or depression.

>> **Anxious-preoccupied attachment.** If you're an anxious-preoccupied attacher, you likely experienced judgment, avoidance, or even ridicule from your caregivers when you expressed a need or showed vulnerability as a child. (Some of your parents' harmful behavior may have been shaped by a highly distressed or hostile context.)

> As an adult, this attachment style may leave you often feeling insecure and worried about your partners' availability and commitment. You may become overly concerned about the relationship and seek constant reassurance. As anxiety and preoccupation escalates, this attachment style can move into toxic surveillance and a cycle of arguments about imagined infidelities or slights. The anxious-preoccupied attacher's biggest worry is to be left alone, and their behavior often alienates their partners, pushing them away.

>> **Dismissive-avoidant attachment.** If you have an avoidant attachment style, you likely experienced something similar to the anxious-preoccupied attachers. Your parent may have been unresponsive or rejecting when you expressed your needs, but as a child, you acted as if that didn't matter to protect yourself. You suppressed your response, and this suppression has followed you into adulthood.

Adults with a dismissive-avoidant attachment style are not comfortable with emotional expressiveness in their partners and also reluctant to expose their vulnerability. You may distance yourself or require a lot of space when emotions run high in your relationships. You likely will have difficulty responding to your partners' stated needs or expressing your own.

» **Disorganized or fearful-avoidant attachment.** If you have disorganized or fearful-avoidant attachment style, your primary caregivers were likely significantly traumatized people, and they passed this trauma onto you with frightening, harmful, and inconsistent behavior.

Accordingly, this attachment style as an adult is often inconsistent and unpredictable. You may yourself have become frightening and harmful to your partners. If that rings true for you, getting help and healing from your childhood attachment wounds is possible. Healing can make it possible to improve your connections in your intimate relationships and also enable you to create limits so that you don't harm yourself or your partners.

Recognizing your adult attachment style

Going through your attachment history can be emotionally taxing. Take your time with your story. Breathe. When you're ready to think about how your attachment history is impacting your present–day relationships, the following exercise can help you connect the dots among the clues in your formative attachment story and your adult challenges.

ACTIVITY

INTEGRATING YOUR INVESTIGATIONS. Work through the following steps and figure out what your childhood attachment clues reveal about your adult attachment style:

1. **Review the two activities My Attachment Story and Attachment Investigation in the section, "Applying Attachment Theory to Kink Play" earlier in this chapter.**

2. **Read the attachment style descriptions in the previous section.**

3. **Think about a recent difficulty you had during a kink interaction, or think about a particularly bad conflict you had with a play partner or lover at any time in your relationship history.**

4. **Ask yourself what you think your actions during this conflict are revealing to you about your attachment style.**

   - If you can't figure out this step, what similarities do you notice when you look at your story and the different attachment style descriptions.

   - If you had to make a guess, ask yourself what attachment style you think best fits you.

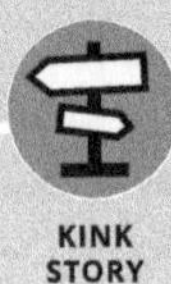

I CAN HAVE THE FEELINGS BUT NOT REACT

I'm just reading about all of this attachment theory in my graduate school program. And it's clear that I'm an anxious-preoccupied attacher — I'm always wondering when the next bad thing is going to happen, waiting for the other shoe to drop.

I don't love attachment theory because most of it is so individualized. In my family, legacies of slavery and ongoing experiences of police violence are so present — what does secure attachment even mean under these systems? My people all raised me knowing that there was a daily likelihood that I could be killed.

And my grandparents have been preparing me for their deaths forever. This is such an echo of slavery — you may have a year or two with your child. They may be sold off when they're ten. These systems disrupted any notion of a secure attachment, and the legacy of those terrors get carried through generation to generation.

The healthy attachment history I do have comes from my grandparents — despite the fact that there was physical violence in the household — really the echoes of slavery — practices that aren't core to our ancestral traditions of childrearing.

So, despite the critique I have of attachment theory and psychology in general for failing to look at systemic violence — looking at the outcomes of disruptive attachment — I thought, well this is info that's helpful. For example, I didn't have an explanation for why I want to be open and live a polyamorous life (see Appendix A) — while I still experience such intense jealousy.

And then I see, oh, literally, I have a father who wasn't around, a mother who would say I'll be back in an hour, drop me at my grandparents, and then would be back in like two weeks. As a result, my agency and autonomy have become very important to me. In my poly life, I feel happiest when I see myself as the center of a group of loving, significant relationships.

Interdependence is a choice — it's the goal. On openness in relationships, I don't want to feel trapped. And yet, sometimes when I experience that agency and autonomy *in others* I'm deeply activated. Mostly I don't know why sometimes when you kiss someone it bothers me and sometimes it doesn't. Maybe I'm just having a bad day. Maybe I feel disconnected or abandoned.

Now that I've got this attachment theory framework I can make different choices around my behavior. I can have the feelings but not necessarily react. There's an explanatory framework there. I'm not broken. Nothing's wrong with me. This intense feeling is partly a result of how I grew up. **—Romeo**

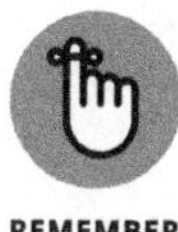

Stop and breathe. You are more than your attachment style. These categories can help you see your challenges and figure out what kind of help you might need. They aren't meant to define or confine you; they're meant to help you take your next steps toward healing and intimacy.

Building Trust Is an Attachment Practice

There's a very old joke about a lost musician on the streets asking a passerby how to get to the legendary performance venue, Carnegie Hall — and the random New Yorker replies: *Practice, practice, practice!*

The same is true about creating vibrant and caring attachments in your kink relationships. How do you get to a place of being ready for intimacy that might activate your attachment wounds? *Building trust in relationships takes practice.*

If your formative attachments involved inconsistency, volatility, or abandonment, you'll need to take some steps to work on your vulnerabilities around trust. Start by owning your anxiety or avoidance about attaching and get some support when your old history is disrupting your kink play or driving you into a state of panic.

Likely you've already had some practice. Perhaps you've noticed patterns in your relationships you've tried to change but keep getting stuck in. Maybe you obsessively chase a particular kink that never works for you. Maybe the opposite happens — your kink *really works* for you and opens you up — but you run away when you get too close to people. Maybe you deflect your partner's requests for intimacy or you cheat on your partner.

The following sections look at your patterns for clues about how your attachment style is playing out in your kink relationships. Here, you can find activities, contributor stories, and reflections that can help you sidestep the fear-driven reactivity that prevents you from connecting with your lovers and find ideas for trying out new trust-building practices.

Reflecting how attachment impacts trust

If you've had a few or several kink crushes or relationships in and outside of the kink context, you likely have a track record that's working for you in some areas, but not in others. Your interest in kink may have been piqued by a sense of hiding yourself, or by disconnects you've had in previous relationships. In this exercise, ask yourself the following questions as you consider your new insights into your possible attachment style and how your formative attachment story may be playing out in your kink attachments.

>> What are some of the recurring problems you've faced in your non-kinky or kink relationships?

>> How have your play partners or lovers described you when they're frustrated or hurt?

>> Does your attachment style explain how some of these problems reoccur?

>> Do you see your issues in a different light when you consider them through the lens of attachment theory and these categories? What insights do you have?

>> What does attachment theory tell you about how you might be sabotaging or hurting your chances at sustaining your kink relationships?

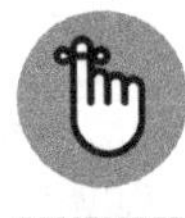

REMEMBER

You're getting a lot of information about yourself in this chapter, which will be extremely helpful; however, you can be making new discoveries about attachment issues that are potentially unsettling.

TIP

Don't be hard on yourself or make snap judgments. Very few people have high security childhood attachment stories or smooth attachment histories as adults.

You can observe your behaviors in the context of attachment theory and identify what your issues are and what you want to do about them.

Aiming for secure-enough attachment

Attachment theory can help you aim for what Jaime calls *secure-enough attachment*. While your attachment wounds may present challenges, you can still move forward and do your best to connect and be intimate with your partners.

You don't have to do this perfectly. You can expect that attachment issues will arise when you're being intimate, especially during kink play that touches the edges of some of your attachment wounds. But you can figure out how to address them together.

So when you're crushing on someone or going on a date with a new kinkster, try the following options to take care of yourself:

>> Talk to one of your besties about how wonderful you are and that you aren't bound by your history.

>> Use a weekly counseling session or support group to dump your anxieties. Let a therapist or your peers hold your anxieties or doubts while you enjoy the sparkly new energy of a crush.

>> Draw on these avenues of support so you can open up to new kink possibilities, rather than stay stuck under the weight of old baggage.

>> Get excited if you've done a lot of work with your attachment story; it doesn't have to define or limit you anymore.

There's nothing wrong with needing support as you step out into new kink possibilities, whether with a new crush or an established lover. Secure-enough attachment doesn't mean your issues will never come up again; it means that you and your play partners accept and work with your attachment histories.

Jaime notes:

In my kink relationships, my best defense against the activation of my anxious attachment responses is to just tell my partners when I feel myself getting into trouble. I may use the Yellow light in the scene (see Chapter 8). And then I may say things like: *I'm getting activated. I need to stop,* or *I have to slow things down and breathe for a minute; my old story is getting in the way.*

> This too, has taken a lot of practice. For many years, I'd get activated with no understanding about what was going on. I was experiencing a kind of terror of being abandoned without realizing it. My heart would race. I'd get lost in a scene or couldn't hear what my play partners were trying to tell me.

> Now I can feel it when my attachment wounds start to get activated. My play partners also know what this looks like because I've shared my attachment history with them and my knowledge about how my attachment anxiety plays out. In my kink family, when anyone notices that I'm deep in my fears — in or out of a scene — they ask, *are you okay?*

> This simple act of care has an immediate, supportive effect. It counteracts what happened when I was a child, when I was definitely not okay, and my parents were unable to be emotionally present and offer comfort. It signals concern for me rather than anger or rejection; it lets me know that the people in my life want to be there for me. I haven't ruined the scene. I can just slow it down. I can stay in the moment and figure out what's going on with me — why am I so fearful or distressed? I can step up to the issue at hand without creating chaos, fighting, or pushing people away.

Developing Communication Pathways That Work for Everyone

Communication practices that work for everyone involve dealing with the partners you actually have, not the ones you imagine. And by that, I mean, here are your kinky beloveds! You've chosen them! They've chosen you! This is miraculous and wonderful and is also bound to come with communication challenges. Embrace them and your different communication and attachment styles. Be committed to improving your own communication skills as best you can. This section provides some straightforward options for assessing your capacity for intimacy and vulnerability as a kinkster. Then, you can start to craft communication pathways that work.

Appreciating and adjusting for differences

The late poet Audre Lorde said that it's not differences that divide people, but the pretense that these differences don't exist. Take this perspective to heart as you analyze communication difficulties with your kink partners. Answer the following questions to figure out your communication roadblocks:

- » Can you adjust your scenes to better suit their needs? For example, always playing in public may be taxing for an introvert.

- » Are you denying your neurodivergence and masking your true ways of being so that you can fit in with neurotypical play partners?

- » Are you having trouble remembering the substance of important consent conversations, leaving your partners distressed when a scene unfolds beyond the boundaries of your agreements?

- » Do you panic when voices are raised during a disagreement? (If you're a person managing PTSD, you may tend to either escalate or abandon the conflict.)

- » Are you judging your kink partner(s) rather than being curious about their attachment challenges and needs?

- » Are you fully aware of your own communication strengths and weaknesses so that you can get to the root of what's not working for you?

Use the questions in this section to make your own self-assessment. Then, you can illuminate rather than deny the attachment styles of your play partners. The questions will help you uncover the roots of conflict and celebrate the great mix of communication strengths and challenges between you and your play partners or lover.

Building the best communication practices

As you build awareness and skill around your communication style and attachment challenges, think carefully about the best forms for engaging with your play partners. Everyone has their favorites.

Here's a simple communication ladder to support good communication:

- **Text:** Is generally best for logistics, keeping up with each other, and getting things in writing — for fast documentation you can refer back to.

  Kinksters love a group chat or text to check in and share parts of the day with each other. Just be sure you don't use it to solve big problems.

  Working out mistakes, breaches of trust, or otherwise highly sensitive subjects by text is the worst. Don't do it.

- **Phone:** If you've made a mistake, or had a communication glitch, get on the phone so your partner can hear your voice and intention and the sincerity of your apology. A phone call is also great for longer exchanges that a text just can't cover, especially to offer comfort to a partner who is struggling.

- **Video:** If you've had a serious breach of boundaries or a mistake that involves a consent agreement, you need to show your face. You need your partner to see the impact of their behavior on you or vice versa. You need to read body language and tone. You need to connect closely to begin a process of repair.

  Alternatively, if you have something wonderful to share or something vulnerable and amazing, make a video call. Share the amazingness.

- **Face-to-face:** All the really big trust and relationship-building conversations should be in person. Did something go wrong in a recent scene? Do you need to change some of your bottom-line agreements? Do you want to start having a deeper relationship, building on your kink connection? Neither text nor phone work for this level of discussion. If you live hundreds or thousands of miles apart, video can work, but only when getting together isn't possible.

A simple way to decide which communication method to use is: The higher the emotional content of a conversation, the closer — vocally, visually, or physically — you need to be to your play partner(s).

Great communication is the basis for every great kink scene. You can always improve as a communicator. Stay open, keep learning, and always appreciate your progress.

Chapter **8**

Creating Safe and Sexy Kink Agreements

Kinksters often engage in activities that simultaneously bring you to the pinnacle of pleasure and to the edge of your physical or emotional limits. How can you ensure each other's safety and well-being in this complex space? In this chapter, we offer well-established tips and tools for co-creating consent and scene agreements that maximize your safety and pleasure. Using these, you can play to your wild, kinky heart's content.

At the chapter's end, you can take all of these great ideas and practices and dream up your own Kink Ten Commandments — what must be present for your kink scenes or relationship to work? Your Kink Ten should let everyone know.

Working with Ground Rules

We have a set of ground rules that we use in every workshop we offer: at work and community meetings, in mediations with partners when things have gone wrong, and in collaborative projects with trusted colleagues. Setting the stage for success by explicitly stating the guidelines or rules for *how you will engage* has never failed to improve outcomes. You can think about whether any of these are useful to you in starting consent conversations.

>> **Use I-statements.** *I-statements* describe where you are at and what you are experiencing. They are entirely self-referential. For example, "That comment was very hard for me to hear because I. . ." is an I-statement. But "I think you're wrong" isn't an I-statement because it's actually a *you-statement* — a judgement about someone else.

>> **Speak one at a time.** This guideline helps to avoid a rush of conflicting voices and interruptions when emotions are escalating.

>> **Listen attentively.** Try to stay out of your head about what you're going to say next and put all your attention on the speaker.

>> **Stay off your phone.** Better yet, agree for everyone to put their phones away to give every person speaking the full attention they deserve.

>> **Avoid speaking when activated.** Generally, you can tell when you're activated because your heart is pounding, and a furious or distressed commentary is flying around in your mind. Wait until you're back in the present, your pulse rate has returned to normal, and you've had a moment to think before you comment or ask a question.

When you're upset at something a partner has said, *call in, don't call out*, meaning you should remember that you respect this person as you present your comment or critique.

>> **Avoid advice-giving.** Instead, prioritize listening, affirming, and asking clarifying questions. If a partner asks for advice, have at it. Unsolicited advice sets you up as an imposed expert on someone else's experience.

>> **Think well of each other.** When a conflict arises, remember the care and hope that brought you here. You have come together to do something extraordinary and out-of-the-box in terms of relationships.

>> **Create time limits for the meeting and for each commentary.** Stick to them. Doing so limits oversharing by the chatty or more extroverted partners. It also ensures that topics or issues are endlessly spinning around ad nauseam.

>> **Making room for tears and laughter raises the spiritual level and collaborative spirit of any meeting.** Adding a guideline that references the way everyone gets through hard things can help set tone.

If you feel that something is missing for you here, add your own ground rule to help set the tone, culture, and intention.

Creating a Consent Container

Creating a container for consent is crucial in kink interactions. Everyone in a kink scenario works together to understand when to start, what the possible tensions or edges of play may be, and where the hard boundaries lie. Most importantly, everyone needs to be clear about what *must not happen.*

Once this container is established, there's room for exploration together — for improvisation, for the spontaneity and wonder of lust and the unknown. The following sections are like a *consent starter-pack:* use the lists and activities to help craft strong consent containers for your relationships or scenes.

Establishing a safeword or gesture

Along with creating your unique roster of likes and dislikes, you'll need to craft a way *to stop all the action instantly* should you find yourself emotionally or physically overwhelmed or endangered in your kink play. *Safewords* and gestures are a hallmark of kink life and culture, as these agreed-upon declarations are the emergency brakes you'll apply in any situation that exceeds your capacity to be present and take care of yourself.

Examples of a situation where you might use a safeword or gesture are:

>> You can't breathe.

>> Your extremities feel numb.

>> You find yourself in a problematic place emotionally.

>> You feel frozen.

>> You feel genuinely afraid, not scared or tenuous in a sexy way.

>> You're doing something you really wanted, but it just doesn't feel right.

   For example, the action or feeling that you wanted to play with — sluttyness or being good/bad, or shame — is taking over the scene in a way that could be harmful, not exciting or sexy. Or you love to play with pain, but on this particular night, the blows that are landing feel harmful, not freeing. Something is off. Or an activity that plays with humiliation or degradation is unfolding in a way that makes you feel actually disregarded or exposed, not the relief or joy that you expected.

>> You can't control yourself emotionally or physically; you're no longer playing within the limits of your agreements.

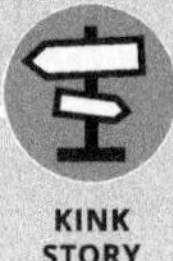

SAFEWORDS CAN BE GOOFY

KINK STORY

For a long time, I had a very goofy partner who really liked comedy. We had seen a TV segment from *The Jay Leno Show,* in which Ross the Intern met the Crocodile Hunter, Steve Irwin. Irwin planned to show him a range of scary animals, and Ross was so scared that he told Irwin he needed a codeword — a kind of safeword. They decided on "pineapple."

So, first Irwin hands him a snake, and he manages to stay calm for a second before using his safeword, "Pineapple!" Next, Steve produces a tarantula, and Ross completely panics and immediately yells, "Pineapple! Pineapple! Pineapple!"

Irwin was like, "Really? Already?"

The whole bit had my partner and I laughing so hard, and from then on "pineapple" was our safeword. It worked for us specifically because it was funny. There were moments in our play when things were very serious or something was going a little too far, but invoking "pineapple" would always make us laugh and bring a bit of humor to the situation because of where it came from for us. **—Robin**

Choosing what to say or do

As you work with safewords and safety protocols, especially while using restraints or a blindfold or gagging your partner, you may need additional ways to tap out should you or your partner find yourselves over your limit. Raising a hand, tapping your partner's body, emitting a particular sound are all great options. Think about what will work, but keep it simple.

Some kinksters love to get creative with their safewords. What's your partner's most hated food? Broccoli could be your safeword. Where's the place you had your worst argument? Marconi Beach could be your safeword. What's your most hated season? Winter could work. The key is to pick a word that instantly resonates but isn't complicated to say.

Respecting the stoplight system

Within the domain of safewords, the stoplight system is much loved for its simplicity and universality because so many people instantly understand the system in the real world. The colors mean the same when you crossing the road:

>> **Red:** Stop *Immediately.*

>> **Yellow:** Proceed with caution, or slow down

>> **Green:** Go-go-go!

The simple utterance of the word *Yellow* or *Red* can turn a potentially injurious moment into a moment of immense pleasure and care.

GREEN MEANS GO

The concept of *affirmative consent,* or checking in when things appear to be going right, to confirm that your partner is enjoying themselves and is perhaps ready for more, is largely a late Millennial/Gen Z addition to the kink theater of engagement. Over time, experimenting with and deploying the Green light has spawned a whole world of kink play in and of itself.

THE MAGIC OF THE YELLOW LIGHT

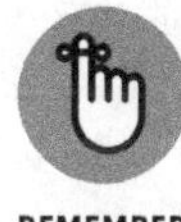

REMEMBER

The Yellow light is the unsung superstar of the stoplight system. While Red appropriately gets a lot of attention, and Green is currently in the spotlight as an innovative tool, Yellow is your best resource and likely most often used light in your kink life.

Do you love pushing yourself with the sexy Dom (Dominant) of your dreams? Be sure to keep your Yellow light at the ready when you find yourself exceeding your limit. Don't hesitate. You are not a cooler or better kinkster by going beyond what you can handle physically or emotionally. In fact, you are the coolest kinkster of them all when you step up and take care of yourself. The Yellow light allows you to slow down the action so you can stay in the scene with your sexy partner. It can give your Dom or Top crucial information to adjust and care for you. A great kink player will receive your Yellow light with enthusiasm and gratitude and change course immediately.

Doms need safewords, too

It's common for safeword discourse to focus on the needs of submissives (subs or bottoms), since they are the people giving up power in a scene, and attention needs to be paid to their limits and safety. But what about their Doms? It's important to remember that every person in a kinky scene has physical and emotional limitations. Each person is responsible for communicating and describing those boundary lines in a consent conversation. And each is responsible for taking care of themselves as a scene unfolds. Sadists, for example, can become overwhelmed by the profound offerings their masochists make. (Chapter 4 has more information about sadism and masochism.) Doms can find themselves activated by their formative stories of abuse and harm, just as deeply as any sub can. Tops can find themselves at the end of their physical limits.

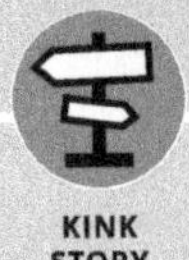

USING MY SAFEWORD MADE ME FEEL LIKE THE BOSS OF THE UNIVERSE

When I was new to kink, I thought the way to show my commitment to the whole enterprise was to be the absolute best at whatever I was doing, and this meant pushing myself, even when I was uncomfortable. This worked for me in my youth as a competitive swimmer. This works for me in my adult life as an employee. So I assumed this was the way to go in my new kink life.

Fortunately, I played with a very skilled Top early in my exploration, who saw what I was doing and called me to account. I learned that my job as a sub was to communicate honestly, in the moment, about what was happening. To reveal and share my experiences, not hide them. This really went against a lot of my conditioning in daily life, where I am often required to stuff my feelings of discomfort or even pain, and to make things work for others.

The first time I used my safeword *Yellow* in a scene, my Dom tenderly praised me and immediately shifted their course of action. It was incredible! Here I am bottoming and yet I hold the power to change things in an instant. *And all that's required to exert this power is to be present in the scene and speak my truth.* I felt like the boss of the universe.
—Jaime

If you are a Dom, respect your own limits. Use your safewords when you need them. If you are a sub or a *switch* (you like to change roles), pay attention to your Dom's condition. Do they seem okay? Fully embracing the two-way nature of consent means tuning into *everyone's* needs in a scene, including the Dom's.

Navigating your consent process

Building a consent container entails choosing your process, content, and documentation. This sounds elaborate, and it can be, if that suits your desires and needs. But building consent can also be relatively simple, especially if you and your partner are experienced at co-creating consent in kink situations. This section provides three options for exploring the consent process with your current or potential partners.

Option 1: A fast discussion

In such a case, possibly as clothes are being removed, you have well-defined bottom lines that you use regularly and are a strong, clear communicator. You are confident that you can read this partner, even if you have only just met.

An excellent consent conversation can be less than a minute long, such as described in the following list (see Appendix A for help with definitions):

>> No penetration, spit in my mouth, I like light restraint and multiple orgasms.

>> Flog me until I cry; sex while I'm crying is a must; aftercare (see Chapter 9) must be at least as long as the scene.

>> Use the stoplight system; anything goes but my left shoulder is sore so no pressure on it.

>> I'm just here to hit you and make out; self-induced orgasms are fine; no touching my genitals; use the stoplight system.

>> I love restraint but nothing elaborate; my safeword is Armageddon; no kissing; you can f*ck me.

Having more time doesn't necessarily mean you will get a better consent agreement than creating one in 90 seconds as you grapple with your partner's clothes and body parts.

The key to a great consent agreement lies in the depth of your self-knowledge plus your capacity to state your desires and limits clearly and to read your partner's cues and needs.

TIP

If you have these tools at your disposal, you can have a perfectly good consent conversation in very little time. If you don't have them, take more time and care when building consent.

Option 2: A quick chat over coffee or a meal

A quick in-person coffee date can be a sweet spot for discussing the consent process. In our case, we are both are experienced kinksters. So when we arrive to the table, we have our lists of YES, NO, MAYBE on our minds or in hand (see later in the chapter). We know what we are after. The coffee date provides an opportunity to assess chemistry and learn whether a new partner has the capacity to listen and learn and take our needs seriously. Maybe you have deal-breaking things on your list like buff arms; long hair; or a loud, unselfconscious laugh. The coffee date or a conversation over a meal can give you all of the essential information in a relatively short period.

Option 3: A getting-to-know-you process

A dear friend of mine loves the slow burn of a long and winding consent-building process — it might be a kink! She enjoys revealing bits of her story over time (days or weeks), offering descriptions of past kink interactions, and building tension in the exchange of past top ten kink experiences among potential playmates. She's an extrovert and loves doing this in person over many meetings; it builds her anticipation and trust.

Perhaps you are an introvert and conversations through e-mail or text is better for you. Having privacy when you are sharing or receiving intimate details may be important to you. Just remember that written exchanges — especially in the sometimes lightning-fast world of texting — can be difficult to read for tone and intent. You have to take extra care with being clear and helping your partner read the mood or temperament behind your revelation. (Emojis can help with this a bit.)

ACTIVITY

YOUR HIGHLIGHT REEL. If you love a slowly unfolding kink conversation, this exercise, which you can also find in Jaime's book, *Great Sex: Mapping Your Desire*, may be for you.

1. **Think about favorite kink and/or sexual experiences to date.**

2. **Pick 3 favorites.**

   Note: In Step 3, you'll be sharing your favorites. If it will be with someone you are very intimate with, you may want to pick the top three highlights from that relationship. If you choose to pick highlights from other sexual encounters or relationships, think carefully about how to do this so that your partner can openly receive this knowledge about you.

   Consider what was happening that made each of these favorites so special. If you prefer, write down the details in a journal, as much as you can remember. Ask yourself:

   - What's alive in you in this situation?

   - If you are with others, what's alive in your partner(s)?

   - Why do you think this experience has stayed in your memory?

   - What would you like to build on or carry forward from these favorite moments or encounters?

3. **Share your highlight reel with someone you are starting a kink consent conversation with.**

   - Share what makes sense given your level of intimacy. Is this someone who knows you well or someone you are just meeting? Share freely and be vulnerable at the level this person has earned.

   - Talk about the happenings and any insight you have for why these experiences are meaningful.

- Be sure to take good care of everyone involved in terms of the level of detail. If you and your partner are in a tender place, for example, perhaps recovering from a breach of trust (see Chapter 12), sticking to highlights between the two of you is probably best.

Sharing your highlight reel can provide important context for a partner you are building a kink consent container with. They can help a potential partner understand the depth and breadth of your kink experiences to date, while finding out what excites you. The sharing session can help each of you get a sense of how easy or difficult it is for you to talk about your desires. And you can get all of that info while having a fun, intimacy-building conversation.

Filling your container

In this section, the focus is on the content of the consent container — what are the things you want to explore? What's inside this nicely bounded container that you want to root around in? The tool in this section gives you many ways to think about how best to fill your container.

With the exception of safewords, there's perhaps nothing more emblematic of kink culture than the YES, NO, MAYBE lists that detail specific kinks and allow you to check off what you are into (YES), what you are shut down or repulsed by (NO), and where you have curiosities or unanswered questions around your sexuality and your kink desires (MAYBE).

These lists are highly recommended and offer wonderfully concrete options for setting boundaries and describing who you are and what you want. People who have never been in kink consent conversations often find the YES, NO, MAYBE lists incredibly liberating. Perhaps you've been discouraged from speaking out loud about a specific desire you have — yet here it is laid out simply and without judgment on this list. Perhaps you've never been able to articulate your boundaries so clearly.

YES, NO, MAYBE lists may have become commonplace or expected in consent-building, but that doesn't make them any less revolutionary or amazing. Find lists that include your favorites or add whatever's missing and go build your sexy, consensual kink life. We provide a YES, NO, MAYBE list in a nearby table.

Classic elements

Some classic elements on a YES, NO, MAYBE list for you to consider:

>> Preferences and limits around sexual activities, such as favorite and prohibited positions, most loved action to give or receive, guidelines around penetration, and so on.

>> Physical vulnerabilities, disabilities, and limits

>> Emotional vulnerabilities, disabilities, and limits

>> Kink activities that drive you insane (in the good way)

>> Kink activities that repulse you (in a bad way)

>> Desires or kinks you have been dying to try out

>> Ways you want to be addressed or attended to

>> Roles you want to take on or avoid

YES, NO, MAYBE lists are often filled out privately and then exchanged by partners who are considering kink play together. If you are an introvert, or a trauma survivor, having a private space to craft and also receive a YES, NO, MAYBE list might be essential to your enjoyment of creating a consent container. In some cases, kinksters find it sexy to interview each other and fill out the lists together. In others, having one person guide the exercise is exhilarating and sexy.

You can do this any way that works for you. Just make sure you are *really checking in with yourself* and answering honestly about what you want — not checking off what you imagine your partner wants from you.

A comprehensive example

Here's a favorite, comprehensive YES, NO, MAYBE list that we created by surveying a number of lists we've used over the years and crafting our own. With a hat tip to Terry Blas and Erika Moen, whose kink list is heavily referenced here.

If any of the terms here are unfamiliar to you, you can find the definitions in Appendix A.

Kinks	YES	NO	MAYBE
Intimacy: Giver=G/Receiver=R			
Romance/affection			
Holding hands			
Hugging			
Kissing			
Spooning			
Pet Names			

Kinks	YES	NO	MAYBE
Sleepovers			
Fuckbuddies			
Friends with Benefits			
Open to loverships			
Public Displays of Affection (PDA)			
Clothing: Self=S/Partner=P			
Clothed sex			
Lingerie			
Heels			
Leather			
Latex			
Rubber			
Uniform			
Military			
Cosplay			
Stripping/disrobing			•
Forced dressing			
Gender play			
Formal clothing			
Steampunk			
Fetishwear			
Clothed/naked dynamic			
Sex Acts and Toys: Giver=G/Receiver=R			
Hand jobs			
Clit fingering			
Blowjobs			
Deep throating			

Kinks	YES	NO	MAYBE
Swallowing			
Facials			
Cunnilingus			
Face-sitting			
Edging			
Teasing			
Mutual or shared masturbation			
Penetration			
Strap-on penetration			
Sex without condoms/barriers			
Tantric/yoni stimulation			
Finger-f*cking			
Object insertion			
Fisting			
Sixty-nining			
Anal penetration			
Anal teasing			
Anal toys/plugging			
Rimming			
Double penetration			
Anal fisting			
Sex in a swing			
Dildos			
Plugs			
Vibrators			
Magic Wands			
Sybians			
Sex machines			

Kinks	YES	NO	MAYBE
Domination/Submission: Initiator or Dom=D/Receiver or Sub=S			
Requiring sexual activities in a scene			
Requiring kink activities in a scene			
Requiring daily activities			
Restricting activities in a scene			
Restricting expression in a scene			
Surveilling daily movements			
Acts of service			
Discipline			
Begging			
Forced orgasm			
Orgasm control			
Orgasm denial			
Role-Play: Top or Giver=G/Sub or Receiver=R			
Glory hole			
Humiliation			
Exhibitionism			
Voyeurism			
Medical			
Human furniture			
Interrogation			
Sleep play			
Hypnotism			
Fake public use			
Practical sex ed			
Puppy play			
Pony play			
Other pet play __________			
Other role-play __________			

Kinks	YES	NO	MAYBE
Taboo/Devastation Play: Giver=G/Receiver=R			
Consensual non-consent/rape play			
Human auctioning/appraisal			
Enslavement play			
War symbolism			
Real public use			
Gangbang			
Kidnapping			
Incest			
Age play			
Surrealist Play: Player=P/Observer or Appreciator=O			
Hentai			
Furry			
Transformation			
Tentacles			
Monster/Beast			
Alien			
Unicorn			
Body Fluids Play: Giver=G/Receiver=R			
Blood			
Watersports			
Scat			
Ejaculate/Cum play			
Sensory Play/Body Parts: Giver=G/Receiver=R			
Genital worship			
Ass worship			
Foot play			
Tickling			

Kinks	YES	NO	MAYBE
Electrostimulation			
Breath play			
Hickies			
Pain and Impact Play: Giver=G/Receiver=R			
Light pain			
Heavy pain			
Nipple clamps			
Clothes pins/zip strips			
Body slapping			
Face slapping			
Spanking			
Caning			
Flogging			
Beating			
Whipping			
Paddling			
Genital slapping			
Genital torture			
Breast torture			
Hot waxing			
Scratching			
Biting			
Burning			
Cutting			
Sounding			
Bruising (short term)			
Marking (longer term)			

YES, NO, MAYBE lists showcase the creativity and expansiveness of the kink process of building consent. Far from a one-and-done, rushed, or awkward transaction, creating a consent container in kink world is often fun and ever-evolving. For many kinksters, consent-building is an elaborate and treasured practice for growing intimacy, trust, and sexual tension. For others, it's just a simple and essential starting point.

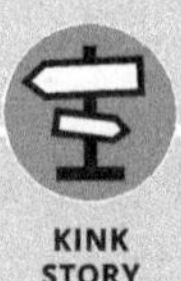

KINK STORY

TAKING OUR TIME TO FIND DIFFERENT AVENUES

I have always been drawn to the Dominatrix role in *BDSM* (see Chapter 4) — a role that gives me a profound sense of control and comfort. When a submissive partner eagerly works to please me, I experience an intense surge of both sexual arousal and power, as if I hold the world in my hands. The thrill of commanding someone while both of us revel in mutual pleasure is simply exhilarating.

However, when I met my partner, she was not into BDSM. For a period of time, she even felt uneasy about my past experiences with it. Because of this, at first, I never fully discussed or explored BDSM with my partner. At times, I even feared that expressing my desires might lead to rejection, which in turn dampened my willingness to explore.

As our intimacy deepened, however, we began to incorporate small elements of exploration into our sex life that she had described as a "maybe" but became a "yes" over time. For example, we role-played a puppy dynamic, where she playfully licked me, and she found it incredibly arousing. Being completely served, worshipped, and attended to during sex gave me that deep sense of satisfaction in a way we both like.
—Ting Ting Wei

MISTAKES WILL BE MADE

Despite your best intentions, and your hard work at being open, honest, and accountable with your kinky partners, at times, things will go badly. Communication will go awry. You will not hear or respond well to what your partner needs. Your kink playmate will miss a step and hurt you. Whichever end of the mistake you are on, it will be painful.

Your value or skill as a kinky partner is not measured by you being perfect, it's measured by how you respond when things go badly. Do you:

You — and nobody else — get to decide the best way to build consent in your kinky life.

An excellent consent co-creation process should feel enlivening, fun, and for some, very sexy. It should give you hope and make you feel safe. If it doesn't, move along. You deserve and can find much more worthy partners.

Creating Contracts

Some kinksters love a good contract. Contracts became famously criticized and memed-to-death after the horrific contract scenes in the much-dissed *Fifty Shades of Gray* movie. Kinky people hated this film! It depicted the opposite of consent: an uncommunicative, self-involved Dom and a deer-in-the-headlights, disempowered sub. It managed to take two incredibly sexy actors and make every interaction between them cringy and repulsive.

Regardless, some kinksters still love a good contract. The creation of them can be wonderfully sexy and creative and provide maximal space for all play partners to stretch into their kinks without worrying about gray areas or misunderstandings. You can create a contract that covers just one scene, a 24/7 experience of kink, or anything in-between. For people with communication styles or brains that really appreciate detail and clarity, the kink contract is for you.

Figure 8-1 is a sample contract you could adapt a zillion different ways to suit your particular kink needs and dynamics.

Sample Kink Contract

_______________________________(Person A/Dom/Sadist/xx's Scene Name)

_______________________________(Person B/Sub/Masochist/yy's Scene Name)

Agree to the following, effective _____________ (Date) to _____________ (Date), at which time this contract will end or be renegotiated. Any participant may also choose to end this contract before that time, for any reason.

Medical considerations. List any medical conditions, disabilities, or medications that might be relevant during play.

Person A: ____

Person B:____

Additional Participants:____

Core safety considerations. List emotional safety considerations and needs, including known vulnerabilities or soft spots.

Person A: ____

Person B: ____

Additional Participants:____

Terms of address. The following names or titles will be used by participants to refer to each other during play

Person A: ____

Person B:____

Additional Participants:____

Safewords and signals.

The following words or signals will be used to stop play immediately:

____

The following words or signals will be used to mean "slow down" or "I'm approaching my limit":

____

The following words or signals will be used to mean "Yes, yes, yes!" or "Keep Going":____

Playing with others. Indicate whether, and under what circumstances, participants may play with others.____

FIGURE 8-1:
Sample
kink contract.

Soft limits. List any acts, scenarios, language, or locations that may cause discomfort and require additional conversation/frequent check-ins:____

Hard limits. List any acts, scenarios, language, or locations that are off-limits and should be avoided during play: ____

Devices and equipment. List devices, toys, equipment, or accessories that may be used during play____

Rituals and routines.

List any special activities that you'll engage in together to initiate a scene:

____

End a scene: ____

Reconnect after time apart:____

Remind each other of your commitment: ____

Other rituals:____

Aftercare. List any activities needed or desired after play has concluded to help participants achieve maximal pleasure and transition back to everyday life.
Person 1: ____

Person 2:____

Dominant/Submissive:
Here's a set of sample Dom/sub directives for a *Dom/sub-specific* contract. In this case, the particular Dom/sub pair enjoys extending the dynamic beyond a single scene, and into public spaces:

Submissive's behavior and responsibilities. The submissive agrees to respect and serve the Dominant, and to abide by the following rules of conduct:
Addressing the dominant as: ____________________Where/when____________________

Mealtimes: ____

Appearance and grooming: ____

Serving the Dominant: ____

Self-pleasure and masturbation: ____

Public conduct: ____

Other: ____

FIGURE 8-1:
(Continued)

Dominant's responsibilities. The Dominant agrees to respect the submissive and act in a way that promotes their health, safety, and wellbeing. The Dominant will be responsible for guiding and training the submissive in the following areas:

Serving the Dominant: ____

Pleasing the Dominant:____

Proper behavior in private and public: ____

Other:____

Punishments and discipline. The submissive will be punished for the following:

Failing to use proper terms of address or disrespecting the Dominant

Punishment(s): ____

____

Violating rules of conduct as outlined above
Punishment(s):____

____

Other Punishment(s): ____

____

Breach of contract. This contract will be considered null and void if:
- Any party ignores or disregards safewords or hard limits.
- Any party fails to discuss/check in before proceeding with an act listed under "soft limits."
- Any party causes lasting harm (physical, psychological, or emotional).

Additional considerations/rules/requests:
____

____

Confidentiality. All parties agree to hold in confidence the terms of this contract unless discussed and agreed upon in advance

Signed

____

Person 1   Date

____

Person 2   Date

____

Additional Participant   Date

FIGURE 8-1: (Continued)

Dreaming Up Your Kinky Ten

Creating your own Kink Ten Commandments can be a way to introduce yourself to potential partners, while building a strong and functional consent container. Your Kinky Ten can look any way you want, and change over time. The list can describe your key kinks as well as any deal-breaking Red lights. Ultimately, your commandments should let your potential play partners know what you want to get out of your kink connections.

Writing out your Kink Ten Commandments can prepare you for any kink consent conversation, whether you decide to share them or not.

If we were writing our Kink Ten Commandments today, here's how they'd look. (Refer to Appendix A for unfamiliar terms.)

Jaime's Kinky Ten:

1. Lies are cheating, in any form. Lies are a deal breaker.
2. Be funny, be kind, and please God, be smart.
3. No sh*t talking about exes or anyone in the community.
4. Tell me stuff you love about your life.
5. I'm a bratty sub who is very challenging to take down.
6. I want you to take me to my most vulnerable spots, but only if you are worthy.
7. I want to take you to your spots.
8. My kinks will morph and adhere to yours, so be responsible with this power.
9. I'm solo poly, so I may fall in love with you, but I won't want to be a partner or girlfriend.
10. In our kink play, let's go where no one has gone before.

Jack's Kinky Ten:

1. If there are things you've always wanted to try but have never had the opportunity, I really want to know what they are.
2. If you start using guilt or shame to try to get more of my time than I'm offering, you'll very quickly stop hearing from me altogether.
3. I welcome sex with all genders and really don't have preferences about genitals.
4. For almost all the kinks I enjoy, I am equally happy giving or taking it, being the Dom or the sub.

5. I love words — verbal, dirty talk, role-play. Potential partners who are also into that jump up the queue fast.

6. I don't mind playing without knowing anything about you (even your name!), but if you then start spewing hate, I will tell you exactly what I think about that and then you will never see me again.

7. If you're very turned on by a kink, it may turn me on too, even if it's not usually high on my list.

8. I like pain — spanking, ball torture, impact play — but my pain tolerance isn't terribly high. If you want to go as far as I can with pain, you have to start small and work your way up.

9. I'm allergic to alcohol, and while I have zero judgment about others drinking, I really don't have sex with people who are drunk.

10. I love to be in bondage, but hoods and other implements that may restrict my breathing make me feel scared in a bad way.

Writing out your Kink Ten Commandments is a grounding exercise that can prepare you for any kink consent conversation, whether you decide to share them or not. And that, we hope, is the big picture take-away; you are the decider in your kinky world of consent-building.

Chapter 9

Developing Great Aftercare Practices

ftercare is an essential aspect of kinky life and for many, a treasured practice. *Aftercare* describes the nurturing and attentive actions you undertake following kink activities that have moved you into an altered or ecstatic state. These activities are so central to a satisfying kink experience that we low-key object to its name because we firmly believe it's a core aspect of kink, not an *after*.

For some kinksters, aftercare is the main event, while for others it's just an important set of closure activities to a scene. In this chapter, you can explore different ways kinksters experience aftercare practices and determine what kind of care you may need after engaging in your favorite kinky activities.

Exploring What Aftercare Delivers

The purpose of aftercare is integration. You and your scene partner or partners may have created an alternate reality together that has shifted your physical and emotional state. During aftercare, you stretch out into the joy and pleasure that your time together has generated and allow yourself to discover whatever is to be learned from this ecstatic intimacy. And then, together, you figure out how to return to yourself and the world around you.

Aftercare is a *cooperative care system*. You work together to come back to the world you left behind during play. If you've co-created a disconnect between your body and your mind, it's about putting yourself back together (more on this in Chapter 10). If you've entered an altered state emotionally, it's about grounding, journeying back to the current moment: to your life of friends, family and responsibilities.

You may find a great aftercare regimen that works for you with one kink partner, and then it doesn't work at all with another. That's because kink is so relational, and the success of any scene hinges on the connection between the two (or more) people, not on a set script that has worked elsewhere.

If you have done a lot of self-reflection and know yourself well, or if you have an extensive intimate or kink history, you'll have crucial information to provide to your scene partners, and this will get poured into the kinky cauldron of connection that you are building together. With these specific-to-you ingredients, you and your partner(s) will be able to create your own unique recipe for aftercare intimacy and pleasure.

Many kinksters report that their aftercare needs change over time. As more of your vulnerabilities and needs are revealed through kink play, your aftercare needs may shift. And, as you age in the scene, what you need emotionally and physically for aftercare may change significantly.

Understanding Why You May Need Aftercare

After a great kink experience, you may find yourself feeling fuzzy, or the world around you may seem out of focus. You may not be able to verbalize what's happening for you. Or you might feel like you have exhausted every energy cell in your body and are completely drained. You might feel like your body is in one place, and your mind is somewhere else entirely, like on another plane or even planet.

Sometimes these states of being are euphoric, other times they are disjointed. They can feel like you are crashing, which is often referred to as a *drop* (see Chapter 10 for more on drops). In any case, these states are brought on when the mix of hormones and feelings that are released by your kink practices are activated at very high levels, and then perhaps depleted.

Our objection to the term "aftercare" is akin to the objection we have about "foreplay." Because foreplay *is sex, dear reader,* not something that happens *before* sex. Let's get into the 21st century on that.

In the 2023 National LGBTQ Women's Community Survey, respondents reported all-over body worship, kissing, and cuddling as their top three favorite sex acts. The question was very clear: what are your favorite sex acts? These answers came from a large group of women (5,002) who have been observed to have more orgasms than women in the general population, also known as their heterosexual counterparts.

So, foreplay *is sex* in the same way that aftercare *is kink*. Aftercare is part and parcel of a holistic kink experience.

Every person's experiences with kink euphoria, exhaustion, or drop are different. There's no one-size-fits-all experience.

TIP

Figuring Out What You Need

People's needs around aftercare vary widely. One kinkster prefers to address aftercare on their own and wants a simple verbal or physical cue that play has ended. Another wants an extended, elaborate set of care steps that involve both their scene partner and others. Yet another kinkster wants to have an intimate, one-to-one aftercare experience that includes sex with their kinky playmate. The following exercise may help you figure out which kinkster you are, and what kind of aftercare you might need.

AFTERCARE DETECTIVE. Think about any intimate experience you have had that was emotionally or physically powerful to take this inventory, regardless of your kink or sexual history. Place yourself back to a time where you felt yourself stretch emotionally when connecting to someone and ask yourself following questions:

ACTIVITY

Question 1: What am I like when I have intense sexual or intimate connections?

Here are a few prompts that may help you to fully recall the experience:

>> What's the environment like? Noisy, calm, dark, sunny, outside, in a basement, and so on.

>> What are you like during this intense activity?

Socially — introverted, extroverted, withdrawn, chatty, silent

Sexually — ferocious, needy, grabby, exhibitionist, aggressive, wanton, shy

Emotionally — weepy, silly, generous, giving, self-focused, other-focused, giggly

>> What's your partner like? Socially, sexually, emotionally?

>> What do you think is the biggest contributor to the intensity of this experience?

Second, remember how you felt:

>> What's happening in your body?

>> If you could describe your emotions in three words, what would they be?

Question 2: What are some great ways that I've taken care of myself in other emotionally intense scenarios?

>> I put in my earbuds and take a hot bath.

>> I call my best friend and talk it out.

>> I climb into fresh sheets, cover myself in quilts, and have a good cry.

>> I take a bike ride to my favorite spot.

>> I make or eat my favorite comfort food.

>> I take Hot Yoga.

>> I sing in the shower, loudly and badly.

Question 3: How does sex fit into the picture when I am in an emotionally vulnerable space?

>> When you look at your sexual history, how do things go when you are in an emotionally vulnerable or volatile state?

>> Is sex a go-to, self-soothing activity in your life, or is it more complicated than that?

For some kinksters, sex is the key driver of their interest in kink; they engage in kink on the path to a sexual conclusion. For others, you need sex and kink to be entirely separate, and sex-as-aftercare would be awful. For others, sex can be a fantastic option as part of an aftercare scenario.

Which kinkster do you imagine you are?

Question 4: Do I tend to ignore my emotional and physical responses during a demanding period like exam week, a break-up, or a death in the family?

If you answered yes to the question above, you'll need help figuring out how to care for yourself in kink spaces — before, during, and after.

If you routinely suppress or ignore your feelings and distance yourself from pain or grief, you'll have a very hard time sifting through your desires when attempting to co-create kinky scenes. You may also find it difficult to identify and articulate what you need in terms of aftercare.

But the good news is, you can use the questions in this activity as a starting place. By being honest with yourself, you can take steps to prepare to relate intimately and safely in kink spaces.

Use the text marked with an Activity icon here and in the remaining chapters in this book and tell yourself the truth. Then you can use the information you've learned about yourself to begin to build a path to the vibrant kink life you want.

STILL LEARNING ABOUT AFTERCARE

I used to think aftercare was mostly for the one who got left with the bite marks — the one who received deserved to be tucked in, fed, kissed, watered. No marks, no aftercare. That was my logic. I built my rituals around being the one who gave: slaps, sensation, attention. I poured my energy into the performance of the scene, assuming that once the play ended, so did the need. Then one day, after a scene that wasn't physically heavy but emotionally deep, my Top looked at me and said, "You never offer me aftercare." It stunned me. I had never considered he might need it. I had centered care around what could be seen, not what could be felt. That realization broke something open in me. Now, I check in. I ask questions. I make space. I think about the emotional intensity of what we co-create — and the softness that follows the charge. And lately, I'm learning be open regardless of the role I'm in. To be held. To be asked. To be under someone else's care, too. I don't always know how to receive it yet. But I'm starting to understand that I need it just as much. **—Tia**

Figuring out when to do aftercare

Aftercare is most commonly discussed as a series of actions you take immediately following a scene. But depending on the kinkster, that may not be the preferred time frame for when care is most needed. Later in this chapter, you can find testimonials from a number of kinksters with greatly varying aftercare needs. Here's a good framework for working out the "when" of aftercare:

>> In the immediate aftermath of a scene, check in with each other. Your pre-scene container creation should have outlined each of your aftercare needs. (See Chapter 8 for more information on creating scene containers.)

>> Determine whether the guidelines were relevant. If needed, the consent agreement can be adjusted for the future scenes.

>> Take care of each other as you've agreed. Is it a phone call the day after? A walk in the park later in the week? Aftercare comes in many forms, in many different time frames.

Connection — understanding the needs of your scene partner — is the most important thing.

REMEMBER

Identifying who does the aftercare

If you are engaging in a scene with a collective group of kinksters, this can be a maximally supportive scenario for aftercare. During heavy bondage, domination, sadistic, or high-impact scenes, the demands on both parties are intense, and while the submissive's (or sub's) need for aftercare may be obvious, the Dom's (or sadist's) needs may also be very significant.

Preparing a Menu for Aftercare

Like all aspects of kink, aftercare is an ever-evolving and expanding universe of practices. Often, aftercare can extend the experience of a scene, while also providing the kind of grounding scene partners need to get back to "real life."

Recently, Jaime watched an incredibly elaborate rope binding and rigging scene that took about two hours, with the sub eventually suspended in the air in a complex set of *shibari* knots (See Appendix A). After the rigger had set their partner back down onto the floor, she took over an hour to undo the knots, carefully checking and patting the skin as she deconstructed each knot and unfurled the ropes. Eventually, she sat her partner up on the mat they were on and offered cold water to drink. The two sat and shared giggles and sweet conversation for another forty minutes.

The scene had so much richness to it: enviable expertise by the rigger, total surrender by the sub, and a beautiful intimate connection in its closure. As an observer, Jaime realized that the aftercare was really the most amazing part. She could see that these two play partners had enormous respect and love for each other.

As they co-created closure for their tender scene, Jaime noted three key basics of aftercare:

>> **Hydration.** The universal aftercare offering to always have cold water on hand.

>> **Body check.** Observing the body for impacts to ensure a partner's well-being.

>> **Affirmation.** Partners check in with each other for connection, care, or love.

The nearby sidebar, "Aftercare Highlights," provides some insight into how many contributors to the book express their aftercare needs, take care of themselves, and care for their kinky loves and play partners.

The moral of the aftercare story is: your best aftercare scenario is entirely yours.

TIP

ACTIVITY

AFTERCARE DISCOVERY. Use the questions in this exercise to determine what you might prefer for aftercare.

Question 1: How do I like to soothe myself?

>> Do I engage in repetitive physical activities that soothe me?

>> Do I have repetitive vocalizations that soothe me?

>> Does laughing (or crying) bring me back to myself?

>> Do I like engaging with loved ones, or do I need alone time?

Question 2: What kind of external or environmental inputs might support my aftercare?

>> Do I prefer music, silence, audiobooks, poetry, visual art, and so on as soothers?

>> What's my favorite kind of soothing touch?

>> What kind of sensations soothe me — a bath, massage, silky fabrics?

>> What kind of food or drink calms and comforts me?

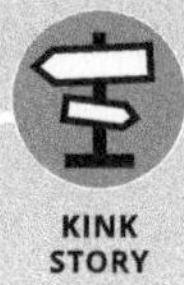

AFTERCARE HIGHLIGHTS

Aftercare is me time: After that evening's scene, I wrapped myself in my fleece robe — its plush softness sliding over my hands and arms before settling on my shoulders and back. I sipped water, delighted, while reaching for snacks. Curling up on the couch, I let the gentle texture of the robe envelop me. I pressed play on a comedy — 'cuz, let's keep it light! And I settled in. There I lay in the dim light laughing, snacking, and hydrating until sated. **—Anna**

The length of time needed fluctuates: I need to be held right after heavy impact play. I don't want to talk. Water. A blanket. I need 100 percent of the attention. Sometimes, my Dom is so exhausted that another dear friend does the aftercare. It's the most perfect part. My body is vibrating, I'm flying, and I want to be surrounded by love. At times I only need 15 minutes of this, others much longer. **—Anonymous**

Aftercare can extend to a few days: One of my favorite aftercare experiences was after a public caning where I was so out of it on the day it happened — in a stratospheric euphoria. I couldn't really connect with my Daddy (see Appendix A), so he came by two days later, and my bruises were crazy — the wild colors, how completely they ranged over my a** and my thighs. He put me over his lap and pressed on each of them, slowly and deliberately. It brought the whole wild event back to us in these tiny flashes of pain; it extended that incredible pleasure. But it also gave us an intimate, private experience of it that I'll always hold sacred. My sadistic Daddy tending to me so gingerly! It grounded us both. **—Jaime**

Aftercare isn't a must: I'm happy to offer it to folks if they want or need it. I don't generally require or ask for aftercare. I do like settling in a hot spring or hot tub the day after I get a good beat down. It really brings my experience back to life in comforting ways. **—Mija**

Aftercare can be an extended process: I took a long walk about four or five miles after bottoming in the bathhouse for the first time. I ended up by the lake. I realized how sore and tired I was after a good hard workout. So then I had a shower, put on some Gospel — I start a lot of meditations in the shower — and washed the night off of me. I was sloughing off a mix of shame, anxiety, and embarrassment. I loved rinsing away the feeling of having my boundaries violated in ways we agreed to because it also washed away residue of times that my boundaries had been dismissed and violated. I put on lotion while affirming everything I loved about the night — the soreness, the feeling of escapism, and pushing my body. And then aftercare extends for me when I debrief with friends for the next week or so. **—Romeo**

Creating long-term traditions in aftercare: Every date would end with the sweetest aftercare. I would give the good boy (Jackson) a bath. It would be so soothing and tender. I would ask him to relax. Let me tend to his body. Let me marvel at his marks or his raw skin. He would drift into a floaty attention. Watching me move and attend to him. I would help him out of the bath. I would dry him off. Help him get ready for bed. I would crawl into bed with him cradling his naked body. I would hold him while he drifted off. I would leave him after a time. I'd pack up my things and head out.

Another aspect of our aftercare dance was via written e-mails the next day or two after the date. It would contain a numbered account of how he felt about our time together. He would recount and debrief the event. Positives and negatives. Things he liked and things he didn't like as much. It was such a beautiful way to connect, receive feedback, and savor our time together. **—Amelie**

Aftercare engages one of his favorite kinks — bondage: I love bondage in all kinds of contexts, but my favorite is *bondage-as-aftercare*. The tighter, the better for me, but anything that removes the element of choice works — from cuffs to a straight-jacket, or my full-body sleep sack. I remember a day when I had just had an excellent heavy impact-play romp with a buddy. We often ended our impact-play sessions with bondage, but we were at a friend's house and didn't have the equipment that we usually used. In order to get me what I needed with the tools at hand, he just laid his body on top of me and let his full weight hold me down. **—Jack**

Aftercare can move into sexy and sexual space: After an intense masochistic scene, I really need to have penetrative sex. It's like the ultimate invasive act for me, the cherry on top of all of the other demands and marking. I want to be f***ed really hard, so that all the vibrations and abrasions on my skin are registered more deeply, inside me. Then, I feel like I'm finished. Completely owned and cared for. If we end an intense scene and I don't have this, I'm much more likely to have a bad drop after. **—Anonymous**

Sex isn't what they need during aftercare: Once I connected with a Dom at a play party for an impact scene. She brought up aftercare and I asked for hugs and cuddles at the party. But she didn't seem to want to stay at the party after the scene, saying that it was too busy for proper aftercare. So, we left. I was still very much in the afterglow of the scene and subspace. She found us a private and quiet room. As soon as the cuddling started, things started escalating. We were suddenly kissing and she started moaning and grinding on me. It was unexpected and uncomfortable. I'd thought we'd be exchanging sweet hugs, and here I was in the middle of a hook-up. I felt robbed of my aftercare and decided to de-escalate the situation. I paused, gave her a hug, and excused myself. **—Aredvi**

What do your responses to the Aftercare Detective exercise (earlier in the chapter) tell you about what you might need? What do your Aftercare Discovery exercise and these testimonies suggest? The only way to truly discover your best aftercare practices is to try them out and communicate your needs to your partner.

Knowing That Aftercare May Not Work

Sometimes despite all your excellent communication and planning, in the aftermath of a great kink scene, you just can't resettle. You may even have had fantastic aftercare following an amazing scene, but then you experience a terrible low a day or two later. You brain is mush. You feel physically sick. Or you're so distracted and forgetful and *not present.* As mentioned earlier in this chapter, this is what is typically referred to as sub or Domdrop (see Chapter 10).

What do you do? Just keep doing what often works. Call your loved ones. Have someone bring you soup. Let your sub or Dom know that you are struggling so they can be of comfort. Let your life partner or bestie know so they can adjust their expectations and offer more care. Drops pass, so keep reaching out for connection. Keep pursuing what you need.

And if your drop hangs on for longer than a week, seek help. You might not be ready for the level of play you are engaging in.

A trained professional can help you sort out what kind of healing work you may need to proceed with the kinky life you seek. At the bare minimum, a good counselor will help you reset your system and set you back on your daily path.

The good news is: kink life and kinky practices anticipate and welcome change. Articulating, observing, listening to, and responding to changes in your relationships, in your scenes, and in the moment are all core tools in the kinky toolbox. Opening yourself to your and your partners' various and changing aftercare needs is part and parcel to a vibrant kink life.

3
Managing Common Challenges

Identify the many emotional states that kink play may evoke and figure out how to deal with them.

Gain skills for encountering your history of harm or trauma while engaging in kink play.

Find tools to deal with common relationship challenges — like jealousy and broken trust — while engaging in kink.

Chapter **10**

Managing Emotional Vulnerability and Risk

Like all forms of intimacy, kink play involves emotional risk and vulnerability. But more so than non-kink intimacy and sex, kinksters report finding themselves cracked open by kinky activities, their most hidden or denied parts of themselves laid bare.

This is part of the mystery and wonder of kinky life. Together with your lovers or play partners, you may engage in sensory or sexual play that reveals your inner self on a deeper level. This experience may release buried memories or frozen parts, freeing you to be more present and grounded in your daily life and relationships.

It makes sense then, that you may want to take extra care in considering how you want to approach these intimate possibilities. In this chapter, you can explore the benefits and risks of delving into the emotionally vulnerable spaces that your kinky exploration may take you to. Do you want to dig deeply into your psyche and your sexuality via kink play? Are you prepared to take care of yourself and your partners when you arrive there? The activities here can help you answer these key questions.

Mixing Sex and Kink

Mixing kink and sex may seem like a no-brainer to you, an organically connected duo. But in kink worlds, the relationship between sex and kink plays out in many different ways:

» For some kinksters, kink and sex are the same thing; each is integral to the other. Kink is an essential aspect of their core sexuality.

» For others, there's a hard line — kink is over here, sex over there. These are two separate worlds of intimacy that may or may not precede or follow each other.

» And for still others, kink is a ultimate form of intimacy in and of itself, period. Many asexual people experience kink this way, as do people of other sexual orientations.

The important thing for you in all of this is to simply take in that one-size does-not-fit-all when it comes to the relationship between sex and kink. You get to decide what yours is. And you should certainly not assume that anyone else has the same relationship.

It's an amazing and beautiful task that is all your own — figuring out the relationship you imagine or desire between sex and kink in your life. And even more importantly, as an experimenting kinkster, you'll need to determine how to manage the vulnerability that kink creates in terms of your emotional and intimate states. That is, you'll need to know if/how you want to engage in sex when you are in those states.

Here are some great questions to ask yourself when you're trying to figure out emotionally whether sex and kink are something you want to mix, and whether you and your play partners are well-prepared to do this.

» Do you enjoy breaking down — screaming, weeping, or forcefully emoting during or after sex? Or do you prefer to be more even-keeled emotionally during sexual encounters?

» Do you have a partner or partners who can take care of you when you're in euphoric or distressed emotional states during sex? If not, are you confident that you can identify such partners?

» Do you feel solid in your abilities to communicate what you're feeling and are able to signal a slow-down or all-stop if sex becomes too overwhelming while you are in a scene?

» How would your partner or partners answer these questions?

Your answers to this brief list of questions can give you good starting points to consider how kink-plus-sex might play out for you.

Identifying Altered States

As you start to manage your emotional well-being on the kink journey, it's important to be aware of the different altered states that kink play can provoke or generate. You can explore these states by reading about them, going to kink demonstrations to observe, or attending a kink dungeon or play party. Afterward, you can experiment with different forms of kink play with a partner and observe your own and their altered states. The following discussion of these various altered psychic states can help you decide what's best for you.

Spacing

Spacing is most often talked about as subspace in kink worlds but Tops (Dominants or Doms) also experience this euphoric state. Generally, *subspace* and *Topspace* describe the woozy, intoxicated feeling of being high on a mix of chemicals/hormones that are released by the intensity of kink play, including adrenaline, cortisol, and endorphins.

When Tops are supporting their subs (submissives or bottoms) in subspace, they may notice them become so altered by their euphoria that they can no longer connect in the present. For example, the sub may become nonverbal. And Tops who find themselves in this spacey high may have to manage being flung out into a stratospheric euphoria while also attending to the well-being of their subs.

You can set various boundaries for when you are in subspace — some bottoms have a no-sex rule while in subspace, while for others, it's their favorite time to be sexual. Tops may set limits around pain-producing activities or Dom practices that require careful attention when they are in Topspace. While, for others, it's serious go-time.

Many kinksters describe Topspace or subspace as flying. But as we all know, what goes up, must come down.

Dropping

Dropping describes the state of having exhausted all the sexy chemicals that have lifted you into blissful space, and how your body and mind feel while running on empty.

While "spacers,"(see previous), are often wobbly and emotive or clingy, droppers might feel cold, teeth chattery, confoundingly depressed, or withdrawn. You may find yourself working with subspace or Topspace in the immediate aftermath of a kink scene, and subdrop or Topdrop hours or days later. You might find yourself working with a drop mid-scene or just as your scene concludes. Staying closely connected to your scene partner, talking with them, taking in visual cues are essential to assessing what kind of state your partners are in and what kind of care or aftercare will support them. (Chapter 9 has more information about aftercare practices.)

Drops are especially responsive to hydration, tender feedback and touch — any kind of attentive cushioning or sheltering of your partner. Of course, every person is different; some kinksters want to be alone during a drop, for example, or don't want to be touched. As always, communication is key.

Dissociation and regression

Dissociation and regression are two states that occur when your anxiety, fear, or euphoria in a scene cause you to split mentally. For example as a sub, you might find yourself "looking down" upon your anxious self from the ceiling. Or as a Top, you might be watching your euphoric self wielding your favorite flogger, while some part of you takes an emotional victory lap around the room. These *dissociative* responses (mentally detaching yourself from what is currently happening) may have developed from surviving a family dynamic that was highly stressful, or having experienced a tremendously boring life at school. If so, dissociating during a kink scene won't be shocking or difficult for you, and you may find ways to take good care of yourself and your partners in a dissociative state. If not, dissociation can feel scary or overwhelming, and you might need to take a time-out.

Similarly, *regression* also involves splitting off from what's happening in the present, but it actually refers to the specific state of moving into and inhabiting a younger version of yourself. When you find yourself in a regressive state in a scene, you may suddenly have a highly idealized relationship with your Top. You may need things that you've not needed before — a kind of attentive care that possibly relates to needs that went unmet when you were a small child or even an infant. This is all good, as long as you feel okay about yourself and the Dom who is caring for you in this state.

TIP

If you find yourself in a space you are not comfortable with, you can use your safeword or signal when you regress (See Chapter 8 for establishing a safeword or gesture). You and your scene partner can create a plan for aftercare in the event of a regression that supports you coming back to your adult self.

Subspace and subdrop are discussed about a million times more often than Topspace and Domdrop, so let's fix that right here. One of our contributors, Anna, is a *switch* (can be Top or a sub). When Jaime asked her what's the difference between how you feel as a Top from how you feel as a sub? She said, *there's no difference.*

And wow. That was a surprise! And while this isn't true for every switch, Anna's response was very instructive and helped us pay better attention to the needs of Tops in writing this chapter. Topspace, like subspace, is an exhilarating and sometimes dissociative state. Domdrop, like subdrop, is what happens when all of those sexy chemicals that fly around when you are at the height of your kink experience have stopped firing, and your body has run out of hormonal gas.

Unlike subs, however, Doms are expected to function well enough to continue to run the scene and attend to the needs of their subs in their altered states. And, depending on the Top, this isn't always possible.

You're not a bad or problematic Dom if you experience drops during or after play. Growing awareness of your needs, owning them, and articulating them to your scene partners is what makes you a great Top.

Flashbacks

Flashbacks are an extreme form of dissociation wherein an event in the present throws you back to a previous — most often traumatic — event. You may get a visual "flash" of the past experience that takes you out of the present and puts you into a highly vulnerable emotional state. You may have significant physical impacts, like freezing or a panic attack. Many people who have experienced flash-backs in a kink scene have learned to either tap out or use a safeword/gesture to alert their scene partners that they need to be attended to. This may also be a way to see if they can continue to stay with the scene.

Only you know what's right for you in the event of a flashback, and a good scene partner will be grateful for your communication about your emotional state. They will take your lead in figuring out how to proceed.

In Chapter 11, we talk more about what it means to play with kink as a trauma survivor, and how to best care for yourself when past traumatic events are re-activated during kink play.

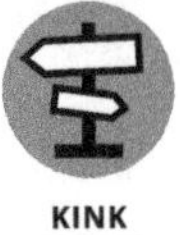

After my mother died, I asked my Top for a heavy flogging scene. I remember holding myself up against the wall in their play space thinking, *why do I even want this?* And they just kept hitting me over and over with a dense, thuddy flogger. Then all of a sudden my mother was everywhere — her final days in our house, sick and vulnerable. Me, trying everything to alleviate her pain. All of the feelings I couldn't have then, because I was in the crisis of managing everything, just came barreling up and I broke down. My Top just gathered me in their arms and let me wail and cry. **—Anonymous**

Holding Space with Care

What does it mean to "hold space" for yourself or others who are in an altered ecstatic or a dissociative state due to kink play? *Holding space* means generously and tenderly extending yourself to the person impacted by centering their care, rather than being in your head, with negative judgments of yourself or them.

Finding your way back

Here are the basics for refocusing while in an altered space:

1. **Take your cues from the affected person.**

   - Check in.

   - Engage.

   - Make sure you have a handle on where your scene partner is at emotionally and physically.

2. **Listen to what is being said *and* read the body.**

   - Take your time, assess carefully — not everyone is verbal in various altered states.

   - Whatever your partner's verbal capacity is, the body also often tells you crucial information.

3. **Breathe.**

   - Everything is better with another breath — your scene partner's physical or emotional state and your reactivity — which will provide the clarity you need in the moment to take the next right action.

4. **Affirm, appreciate, clarify.**

   - Don't: criticize, distance, or deny.

   - If you are worried that you don't have the capacity to affirm, appreciate, or ask clarifying questions of your scene partner when they are in an altered state, use your safeword.

- Then, figure out what you need to do next. You may need to take more time to observe others caring for their partners, or go to workshops at kink conferences, or ask your friends. You can always build your capacity to hold space over time.

5. **Enjoy, delight, celebrate.**

    - Be present for your scene partner and let them know how amazing they are. Rather than: panic or shut down.

    - Again, If you're not sure about your capacity, don't despair. There are so many opportunities to learn and grow in kink community.

Using signals when you can't speak

If you find yourself in an altered state where you are nonverbal or so dissociated you can't continue, the good news is, you will likely have a predetermined way to signal your partner that you need to stop, or slow down. Depending on the activities you are engaged in, one of the following may work for you

- » double tapping their chest, or

- » dropping to the ground

If you haven't created a predetermined gesture and find yourself in a new emotional or psychic territory, you can just signal in any way you can. Here are a few steps you can do to find your way back to yourself:

1. **Look your scene partner in the eye so you can communicate physically that you are in uncharted territory.**

2. **Breathe in deeply and try to lengthen your exhale.** Do this a few times.

3. **Bring your hand to your chest and massage gently at the center.** This gesture is grounding for you and may signal to your scene partner that something is up.

4. **Look around the room and let your eye land on a few solid objects and name them to yourself in your mind:** chair, lamp, table, water pitcher.

5. **Keep breathing.** If you start to feel more integrated, use a safeword to slow down or stop the action.

6. **Repeat these steps.**

Developing a practice of re-integration can take time, which is why planning ahead for dissociative or regressive responses is a great idea.

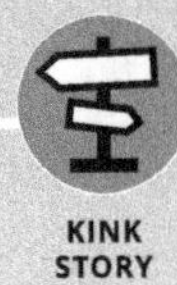

TAKING ON DIFFERENT ROLES

If you are familiar with kink vocabulary, you may have heard about "Topping," "bottoming," "switching" or "being in service" among other roles in the scene. Here's an introduction into the kinds of activities and emotional spaces that people who take on various roles engage in.

Everything isn't for everybody. But in kink worlds, you have the opportunity to experiment with a vast menu of sexy, interesting, creative roles and emotional states. (See Appendix A for unfamiliar definitions.)

Topping: I feel much more vulnerable while Topping in any kind of format. I think this is because I still worry that I am doing it wrong or that I will miss an important cue from my bottom. Especially if it is loud or busy around us. With bottoming, it is about how much I can take, what can I handle, and it helps to always know that in the end, I am really basically in control. Topping feels a bit more like a performance and a test of my creative capabilities. Can I create this scene well? Can I give my bottom what they want? Can I read all the nonverbal cues and body language to intuit if what I am doing feels good or is too much for the person? I feel so much more pressure with Topping and that makes me feel vulnerable. **—Robin**

Bottoming: I have lived with daily or weekly pain and have had to go to the hospital for years. I had encountered medical-setting kinks through a partner and had always felt repulsed, associating it with pain and condescension and misgendering and long waits in the ER and the faint smell of pee. Then I was advised to go to a pelvic floor physical therapist, and I scheduled a series of appointments over Telehealth.

The practitioner recorded her voice directing me what to do so I could self-administer electroshocks through a TENS system hooked up to exterior parts of my pelvis. It did hurt but it also felt good. I felt myself more and more aroused as I turned up the shocks. Exciting images of Dom doctors in lab coats and rubber gloves filled my mind. I thought: "Am I alchemizing my medical trauma into a kink?"

Since then, a robust medical kink has continued to flourish for me, involving role-play with partners. In these scenes, I get to be a sub who gets *experimented on to try to cure my incurable disease.* This play has helped transform my shame as a captive to the medical system as a person with chronic pain into something of my own, something I can grieve and laugh at through being submissive. **—E.T.**

Switching: Being a switch as a trans person who is also genderfluid has helped me form deeper connections and understanding of the different aspects of my gender and myself. Bottoming allowed me to engage in things that were previously taboo for me before transition, such as submission and giving up power and control. I even found that when I find myself in a high femme mood, I become a pillow princess and only want to bottom! On the flip side, Topping in kink has helped me better understand multiple areas of myself. When I Top as a sadist, I often tap into a badass, hard femme side of myself that takes power to please herself. By exploring these, I've come into a much more whole sense of myself as a person. **—Mallory**

Serving: I usually Top, and the only person I've done service with is C., and he's aware that this is very hard for me to do, and that I'm going to be very sensitive to f*cking up, very sensitive to feeling a sense of shame or inadequacy. So, he would start with small things like, what is the predicament you want to define? What is it you think you could do? And then — okay, I'm not telling you that's what you're doing. I will pick what I'm having you do now that you've told me what you're up for.

So, there's almost an interview process. What do you think will be easy about this, and what do you think will be hard?

And I think we've had such a long relationship as equals that energetically, I trusted him when he told me he wanted to try this. It was a way to give him a space that was different from what he had with other people. So, it's about moving into a really different space for me, but also, yes, about him. **—Amelie**

Taking pain: My life as a Top, sadist, and Dom is hot, fun, and fulfilling. But another space I treasure is being suspended with flesh hooks. After losing my Mom and younger sister, I never fully processed my grief. Hook suspension gave me the opportunity for the breakthrough I needed. Alone in the air, with only the pain and my emotions, healing began. I screamed, cried, and released years of sorrow. I saw the ends of the universe, found peace, and came back whole.

Any time I'm doing an energy pull or flesh hook suspension, that's when I'm the most emotionally vulnerable. It's visible, palpable, and afterward, I need alone time to process. Don't talk to me, touch me, or engage until I'm ready. I tell the piercing team in advance, and my partners and friends are great at giving me that space. **—Naria**

Being bound: I haven't ever had a bad bondage experience, but I've also been very picky about who I've done it with. The number is fewer than ten, which is the opposite of how I have approached sourcing partners for other kinds of play where I'm pretty curious and interested in just about anyone. I have to be with someone I really trust because there is often an initial moment when things could go awry mentally. Obviously, I will already have consented to being restrained, but there's a moment when the reality hits my nervous system and everything seizes up a little bit. Sometimes I thrash about, even just slightly, coming to understand the specifics of how tight everything is and exactly how much I can move, and it can feel like there's a moment of rebellion when I want to push against the restrictions. But even as a person with chronic anxiety, that moment has never turned into a panic attack. This is very much because the Doms I'm with have always been people I have such strong positive feelings toward. **—Jack**

TIP

Talking through your hopes, fears, and aspirations with your scene partner in advance of play will help prepare you for all the mystery, magic, and emotional anarchy that your kink connections may create.

Resisting the Critics

Kink destroys categories. It breaks through ideas you have about yourself. It wrecks logical, neat descriptions you have for who you are and how you live in the world. This can be wildly liberating for kinksters. And, for many, it can be incredibly disorienting and difficult. You may have to rethink your identity and your friendships. What matters the most to you in a partner, a friend, a social circle, and your intimate life — all of it might change.

To open yourself to your kink desire, to claim it, often involves resisting a lot of authoritative structures and institutions that have been organizing your life — your parents' view of you, gender expectations in the world, ways of being in your social group, your physical style or presentation, your cultural or religious traditions. Name an arena, and kink can be a big disruptor.

The sometimes-monumental shifts you may experience via kink play can extend to only scenes and the kinky rooms you enter. Or, the impact of your kink exploration can have a much bigger footprint, creating major shifts in your daily life and world. Either way — *that is a lot of emotional territory to cover and manage.*

In this section, we run through some of the big overarching themes about what is considered "normal," which can make it very challenging for you to embrace and explore your kinky wants and needs.

Resisting conformity and the violence of "normal"

Here's a list of several constraining themes of normal that kink disrupts:

>> **Masculinity.** Normative ideas about masculinity tell you that you have to be in charge of everything, especially women you are intimate with. Certainly, real men don't hang with women who drag you around a kink party on a leash or have multiple scene partners.

Real men have to front that you are in charge, not emotional, don't cry, are a primary provider for your unit, and can keep everyone in your intimate life "in line."

By contrast, masculine-identified people in kink worlds may bottom, cry, wail, scream, lose control in a public kink space, submit to people of all genders, and prize others' leadership depending on their partners and situations. They may also be amazing Tops, if that's what their thing is!

>> **Femininity.** As a counterpoint to masculinity, constraining ideas around femininity direct women to be passive, silent about their needs, and devoid of lust or passion. If you've been schooled in this kind of femininity, you might find it very difficult to center yourself in kink play, which is essential for any person co-creating a scene.

Moreover, since girls and women experience sexual coercion and violence at such high rates in the U.S., you may also have to deal with the reality that some of your experiences of intimacy have been dangerous or harmful at some points in your life. You'll have to sift out your desires to play with the edges of what is comfortable or "safe" in your kink life, while possibly navigating the remnants of past harms in your psyche and your body. All while rejecting the idea that you should be silent or accommodating to your partners about what you actually want.

>> **Heterosexuality.** As a system, heterosexuality relies on and perpetuates strict codes around masculinity and femininity. Inside this theme there are very tight rules, For example, monogamy is the only meaningful way to have a relationship; prioritizing pleasure in your life will lead to your ruin; people who play with domination or bondage or pain, and so on, are sick. For men and masculine people, being in control of your family unit is a primary mandate. For women and femmes, submitting and keeping yourself and your children under control is a core directive.

And within this system, there are very strict rules about "appropriate" ways to relate intimately with people who share your gender. These rules are often broken in kink spaces, where watching others play, attending to friends in a scene, or joining play constructed by others often runs counter to dominant constraints around gender and sexual orientation.

Given that kink is often about anarchic relations and a loss of control, it fundamentally disrupts core tenets of heterosexuality.

>> **Queer and Trans Identity.** Because queerness and transness are targeted as wrong by so many different structures of authority — the family, religious orders, the state — there can be enormous pressure to appear to be a "good" queer or trans person to larger society. There's pressure to prove yourself worthy of your right to exist and have a "safe" place in "polite" society. Accordingly, queer and trans kinksters may struggle with their desires. Pursuing kink desire seems like a dangerous enterprise given how heavily the deck is stacked against you. Perhaps this adds to kink's attraction? In a world bent on excluding you, why not go all the way out on that limb? Queer and trans kinksters may struggle with this fraught, contradictory emotional space.

» **Monogamy.** The monogamy imperative says: monogamy is the only functional and legitimate relationship form. Everything else is fake, immoral, or destructive. While you can certainly live a monogamous life as a kinkster, being kinky knocks up against monogamous tenets by placing you in the company of people who have multiple scene partners or who play casually with kinksters beyond their primary relationship. This can be disruptive and scary for people whose social and intimate lives have been centered on monogamous coupledom.

» **Racial identity.** People of color in the U.S. are often targeted and criminalized. They are vastly over-represented in systems of punishment and incarceration and much more often subjected to state intrusion on their families and in everyday life than their white peers. Accordingly, playing with kink may feel like a risky indulgence if you are a BIPOC person. You may have to navigate legitimate fears as you consider stepping into your power and pleasure in kinky worlds. Moreover, you may experience judgment about kink from within your BIPOC families or communities, which is undoubtedly difficult given the hostile state of the world. Despite these risks, BIPOC kinksters have led the way in many communities, historically and in the present. (You can find more about these leaders in Chapters 18 and 19.)

» **Culture and religion.** Your cultural and religious backgrounds may be an important foundation for your life. Your extended family, traditions, and rituals may be an enormous comfort and a significant part of your identity. Kink can run counter to the traditions and religious practices you grew up with. You may find it necessary to hide this part of your life from your family or religious community to maintain close ties that are meaningful to you. A lot of kinksters struggle with this, and many come to a workable solution — a way to live with these tensions. (You can find more about this in Chapter 14.)

As Kinsey and other sexuality researchers have found (see Chapter 6), there really is no normal when it comes to desire and connection. Another way to say this is: what has been sold to you as "normal" doesn't reflect how people in the U.S. and around the world actually engage intimately.

IT'S NOT ABOUT ANYONE ELSE

What sustains my connection to kink — is my own curiosity. I don't rely on other inputs. I'm not really driven by other people's interests. I'm more curious about my own mind and desires. But then depending on how the rest of my life is going, that can be good or bad. I have to have enough order and peace to access it. There's a level of spaciousness I need to have the curiosity. **—M'Bwende**

Use the exercises and information in this book to create an intimate and sexual life that is meaningful to you.

Building a foundation for wellness

Kinksters love to set limits and then break them. As you co-create scene containers with your play partners and fully discuss your kinky YES, NO, MAYBE lists (see Chapters 3 and 8), you may feel differently about what you have defined as a hell-yes or as off-limits once you're actually in a scene. The wonder of kink life is that there are endless revelations and surprises. This is the core function of kink lists: to name where you are, as a launching point, so you can discover where else you may like to go. And every time you find yourself in new, uncharted territory with your kink play, you have to manage your emotional vulnerability.

Building a foundation for wellness in your kink life means establishing a set of practices both in your scenes and in your life that ground you so that you can keep growing and expanding your kink practices. You can maximize the breathtaking intimacy and connection that kink life provides, without harming yourself or your scene partners.

Amelie notes in her following story that this means being really clear about what you can and cannot offer, so you can be fully present for each other emotionally.

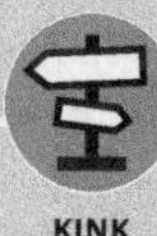

KINK STORY

TAKING CARE OF BOTH OF US

One of my lovers, J., has an attachment wound about his mom not being emotionally present when he was very ill and sick as a young person after his parents divorced. So, he has these memories of being ill on the couch, and she's either very distracted or just not there. And when we got together, I was in this very intense time of parenting and running a business; I literally only had five hours of in-person time to spend with him each month.

To deepen our connection to each other, I'd make assignments for him to write about his desires and what he wanted in terms of kink play as well as write debriefs of what it felt like after time together. This extended our pleasure and helped him cope with feeling far away from me.

He'd often fall into this vulnerable little boy space after hard impact play and sex, and he'd not be able to talk much — just like literally floating. I'd draw him a bath, clean him up, and then tuck him into bed. And then me holding him really helped him deal with

(continued)

(continued)

feeling sad that I wasn't spending the night because that was certainly something that he had never had with a lover before — like *you're actually leaving?* Because of work and my kids, I needed to get home.

And it turns out, that was deeply healing for him and also healing for me; I could be an attentive Top and parent figure and just meet his needs, even within a limited time frame. And it worked. It met a need of his — of really listening to his wants, and being present and coming through. And it met a need of mine too — of really being a good, loving parent who could meet his needs perfectly. At the time, my kids were teenagers, and I was getting so much "feedback" at home, so much criticism and so much *No*. Our dynamic really speaks to the holistic power of kink. **—Amelie**

And finally in the following story, Elisabeth notes that the structure of her life beyond the scenes she's engaged in make it possible for her to experiment and take risks. But not everyone has a supportive life structure beyond their kink life. In fact, many kinksters are escaping oppressive conditions in their daily lives through kink, so navigating how deep to go, and figuring out how to get the aftercare you need may be a lot harder:

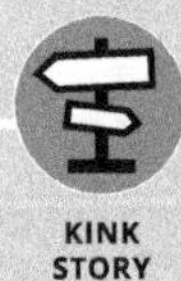

FINDING THE RIGHT POST-SCENE MIX

Coming down from these things — that's something that I have a lot of experience with across many decades and contexts. And I've noticed over the long haul, even since my 20s, that I do very well, because people talk about dropping, say, after parties. And I started realizing at some point — I don't really experience drops.

I started wondering "why"? And I realized it's because of things like, I have my 12-step program. And, I don't have to hide — I'm not leading some kind of a double life which is a huge privilege. I'm not going out and living my fantasies and then coming back to a life and community and people that are totally dissatisfying to me, right?

I don't have to try to cram it all in. There are few expectations on me when I return. And I respect my physical and mental limits. These things seem kind of basic, but they can really make or break the post-scene experience.

It's kind of like you're responsible for your own aftercare. Which doesn't mean that you can't ask for things, but your play partners might not get them right. You have to know that it might not work out exactly the way you want.

Your emotional wellness is your job in your kink life. Your wonderful subs and fantastic Doms can extend superlative care to you in and out of scenes. But if you are not capable of identifying or articulating your needs and vulnerabilities in order to build the best possible conditions for play, you're going to struggle.

TIP

Take your time building self-awareness with your kink practices so that you are giving yourself the space to learn as you go. *There's no rush.* You can have the kink life you want; we promise.

Chapter **11**

Navigating Kink as a Trauma Survivor

Trauma survivors often deal with stigma and naysayers when exploring intimate relationships, as though your experience of harm disqualifies you from the possibilities and joys of sex and connection.

If you're a trauma survivor considering kink, here's the good news: Like all people, you as a survivor are capable of intimacy and expressing your sexuality on your own terms. The nature of your trauma and how much support you've been able to gather to pursue healing will impact your capacity for being vulnerable and close in sexual and kink situations.

In this chapter, you can explore how survivors of emotional, physical, and sexual trauma think about and engage in kinky relationships. The stories, tips, and tools here can help you consider where you are on your healing journey as it relates to navigating kink intimacies.

Because kink often involves moving through altered psychological states, it has healing potential for trauma survivors. Survivors often create or rely on altered states to endure their abuse, press on, and heal.

REMEMBER

Understanding How Trauma Impacts Your Life

All of us survive negative experiences at some point in our lives. *Trauma* is a term that describes what happens in your body and your psyche when these experiences are so overwhelming that you cannot fully process them in the moment. Traumatic experiences dig in, like a psychic splinter, and take up residence in your body in ways you cannot predict or control.

Post-traumatic stress disorder (PTSD) refers to the intrusive and unpredictable ways that present-day experiences connect to and activate an emotional or embodied response to traumatic events in your past. For many who have survived negative experiences that endangered their lives — like war, a car accident, rape, or physical assault — and those who have survived negative experiences that have shattered your sense of safety — such as forced displacement from your home or country, getting fired from a job, confronting a stalker, or leaving an abusive partner — your body and mind may have locked down these traumatic events and stored them away to help you get through the period of crisis.

However, the legacy of trauma and whatever you have yet to process lives on in the ways you interact with others and build your life, especially with your intimate partners. Since your closest friends and lovers are the people you take emotional risks with, they are often the people who encounter your traumatic history. It seems incongruous or illogical that the internal territories where your deep trust, joy, and ecstasy live are often pressed up against or situated atop your stored pain and terror. But there you have it. Stepping up to love, stretching your emotional capacity, and being vulnerable and open – all of these incredible, wonderful pathways to growth can be littered with traumatic potholes from the past.

The following sections will help you sift through the specifics of surviving traumatic formative and adult experiences so you can start to consider how these might be impacting your present-day ability to express your needs and navigate conflict in kink relationships. (To look deeper at attachment theory and issues specifically, Chapter 10 presents key information for you to explore.)

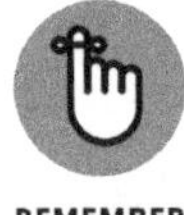

REMEMBER

An important term we use often in this chapter is *activation.* When trauma survivors experience an event in the present that mimics, recalls, or connects to a past event that involved abuse or harm, a trigger response can be *activated* as a result. When you're activated, you're no longer responding to the present situation. Instead, you're in survival mode, which often features an outsized panic response of fighting, disappearing, becoming frozen, apologizing for yourself, or overly attending to the person who has set off the trigger. This response is called fight, flight, freeze, or fawn (discussed in Chapter 7).

Being a good communicator means knowing how to inform your partners about what's happening in your body, brain, and heart. Then, you can take a break, if needed, and eventually move from a traumatic activation back into the present.

Looking at your ACE score

In the mid-80s, an obesity researcher and treatment specialist became frustrated with his poor results. Dr. Vincent Felitti found that no matter how much education he provided his patients around nutrition and behavioral modification, they didn't sustain weight loss. He decided to interview his patients to see if he was missing anything important and was shocked by what he found: a very high percentage of his patients had experienced childhood sexual abuse.

This finding was the starting point of an extensive arena for study — adverse childhood experiences (ACEs) — and the creation of ACE scores by Felliti and his research partner Dr. Robert Anda, which calculate the load of adverse experiences on a child's formative years. These researchers were shocked to find a direct connection between high ACE scores and adult disease and mental health issues. Children with an ACE score of 4 or higher, for example, were found to be more likely to suffer from chronic bronchitis, emphysema, stroke, or heart disease as adults. High ACE scores are also associated with higher rates of alcoholism and drug addiction, and, as Dr. Felitti observed when he started — obesity.

What does the ACE measure? The ten key experiences that make up the score are listed here. Each experience is assigned one point.

>> Did you experience frequent emotional or verbal abuse by a parent, including put-downs, humiliation, and threats?

>> Did you experience frequent physical abuse by a parent or other adult, including pushing, grabbing, slapping, or throwing objects?

>> Did you experience sexual abuse by someone five years or more older than you in your household, including a parent or sibling, including touching, fondling, or penetrative sex?

>> Did you experience emotional abandonment? Were you on your own emotionally? Did no one care for you or have your back?

>> Did you experience economic hardship? Did you not have enough food or clothes? Did no one protect you? Did you not go to the doctor when you were sick?

>> Did you experience divorce or breakup between your parents?

>> Did you witness violence against your mother or stepmother?

>> Did one or more of your parents drink or drug excessively?

>> Did one or more of your parents have a mental illness that impacted you?

>> Did one or more of your parents go to jail?

Many researchers have built on Felitti and Anda's work, which although imperfect, has established a highly impactful field of inquiry. In the years following the development of the original ten questions, researchers have noted that divorce in itself isn't necessarily a bad experience for children, depending on how the parents manage it. And the construction of the sexual abuse question isn't great — many people survive sexual abuse from siblings less than 5 years older than them. The questions miss witnessing violence against siblings, and they entirely miss sexual abuse from people not living in the household. Other researchers added a longer list of concerns to measure, such as experiencing frequent housing displacement, being in foster care or having your family surveilled by the child welfare system, and being exposed to police violence.

Nonetheless, even without these improvements, the original ACE measurement provides crucial information for anyone trying to measure their exposure to traumatic experiences in their formative years.

FINDING YOUR WAY THROUGH THE PAIN

Perhaps you've never considered how your childhood experiences influence your adult attachment patterns. If so, this territory can be fraught, and that's okay.

Take your time with this information. If you survived any of the brutal or disruptive events that are described in the "Looking at your ACE score" section, the good news is that those experiences are over. You are an adult. You can decide how you want to relate to your history of trauma or abuse. If you're like us, sorting them out may take years.

Today, there's a great deal more understanding about the prevalence of emotional, physical, and sexual abuse in childhood. According to the Centers for Disease Control (U.S.), 1 in 4 girls and 1 in 6 boys experience sexual assault before the age of 18, and this prevalence is higher for LGBTQ+ and BIPOC girls. The prevalence of emotional abuse in childhood is much higher, across all genders, and is often reported as between 36 and 44 percent.

And research has largely contradicted the idea of a stranger as most likely to commit these abuses. Most sexual abuse is committed by people known to the survivor;

emotional abuse of children is most often perpetrated by a family member; teen assaults are most often committed by friends and romantic partners. Great advances have been made in understanding and treating childhood trauma, while also understanding that it leaves the survivor at risk for abuse in adulthood.

Although treatment for trauma has improved tremendously since our childhoods, finding appropriate healing resources, acceptance, and good love can still be a difficult road. If that has been true for you, you're in good company. Healing from trauma is a lifelong process. The work gets a lot easier when you find others who share similar experiences. In community with other survivors, recognizing and appreciating the sacredness of your survivor journey is often easier.

Connecting the dots between your past and present

Making connections between your childhood emotional, physical, or sexual abuse and the reactivity you may feel with your scene partners or kinky lovers is crucial to a safe and pleasurable kink experience. Sometimes, activation occurs within a scene. Sometimes it comes after kink play, when you have perhaps found yourself in uncharted emotional territory.

What can you do when you find yourself activated by kinky ways of relating that you love and want to pursue? The following exercise can be used as is as an important tool to help you figure out the best ways to build constructive kink connections while healing from past experiences.

ACTIVITY

TRACKING AND DE-ESCALATING YOUR TRAUMA RESPONSE. You'll need a sheet of paper (or journal) to write down the following headings to create a chart to track your activations.

>> Date

>> Activity

>> How I Reacted

>> Origin or Parallel

>> Care/De-escalation

You can fill in the chart when you find yourself in a reactive space with a lover or scene partner around past trauma.

As an example, the Table 11-1 details the triggering behaviors that a fictional kinkster, Kendra, has identified in various kink and everyday scenarios. In each of the entries, Kendra noted her reactive responses, and what steps she (and in some cases, her scene partners) took to de-escalate her emotional state and take care of herself.

TABLE 11-1   ## Tracking Your Trauma

Date	Activity	How I Reacted	Origin or Parallel	Care/De-escalation
2/5	Worked on the scene container for a new scene with Bill	Got agitated and shut down	Bill was overly directive, and I fell silent in the way I did with my abusive boyfriend when he took over discussion.	When I got home, I called Bill and let him know I shut down during our meeting. He asked me what he could do to take care of me.
2/29	Went to the Sunday morning Kink Munch	Had to leave the table because I had a panic attack	J. and E. were arguing over who should pay the bill, and I flashed back to my father's abuse after any public family conflicts that embarrassed him.	S. came to find me in the bathroom and helped me get grounded and regain my breath. J. and E. gave me hugs and showed me that they were not upset with each other or with me.
3/12	Flogging scene at the Playhouse	Broke down early in the scene	Usually, I love the rhythmic thudding on my shoulders, but this time I flashed back to my mother beating me with a belt.	T. stopped immediately and held me, saying "I'm right here, I've got you" over and over while I cried. T. brought in P. and E. for extra support during aftercare.
6/3	Bondage scene	Felt terrified when Dom (my Dominant) put the hood on me at the beginning of the scene	When I was punished as a child, I was often left on my own in darkness.	J. talked to me and stroked my arms as we had planned. Her voice and her touch were steadying, and then we were able to continue and had a hot, sexy scene together.

REMEMBER

De-escalation is a practice encouraged by therapists, body workers, and somatic practitioners so that clients can come out of a state of *activation* and return to the present moment. Breathing and spotting/naming multiple objects in one's field of vision are common de-escalation techniques.

You can see from this table that Kendra is at a place in her healing process where she's activated fairly often by certain kink scenes and a partner's behavior. But the good news is, she's done a lot of work on her trauma history. Kendra has a great deal of insight about the sources of her activation and the kind of care she needs when she finds herself thrown back in time to past events. She also has amazing kinky loved ones around her who are responsive and kind.

Although you might not know much about your history yet or be able to identify what activates your panic or shuts you down, you can work on identifying action steps that can help you come back to the present to feel grounded and connected with your partner. (See Chapter 9 for great aftercare practices.)

When you understand your story on a deeper level and can identify your triggers, you are on a path to developing ways to reconnect to the present and communicate with your partners. Like Kendra, you can begin to heal even from multiple traumatic events.

When you create your own chart, don't be too hard on yourself if you find that you're getting activated a lot. Instead, appreciate the level of emotional strain you may be carrying into your kink scenes and relationships.

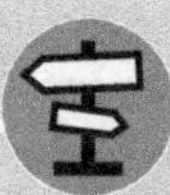
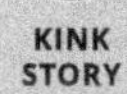

I CAN SEE THE HARM AND GET SUPPORT

I was super activated once at a big kink conference. I went back to my room and called my friend IG, and we really talked it through. I mean — I was triggered to the point where I thought the Dom might follow me back to my room. I put a chair against the door. The beauty of my friendship with IG is that we talked through all the things that went wrong in the interaction. The Dom was definitely at fault; they didn't listen well to my boundaries or read my responses. But after talking with IG, I realized that I was upset with myself, with steps I took and didn't take in the interaction. It helped me focus back on me and my own agency. It totally de-escalated my fear and distress. So much so that the next day when the Dom checked in and asked if there was anything I needed to talk about, I could honestly say no — I really didn't need to talk with them. I had gotten a lot of information from the scene around how I needed to take care of myself in the future, and it really wasn't anything I wanted to talk about with them. They were not someone who was going to be an ongoing part of my life or my kinky world. And in a lot of ways, my learnings from the scene were not for or about them. They were for me. I was totally able to move forward. Yes, the interaction was harmful, but it actually wasn't traumatizing, because after the harm — I was able to access help — my community. **—Aredvi**

De-escalating Your Responses

This section focuses on de-escalation or working to contain or lighten a past-trauma-induced, crisis-level response to a present-day situation. The checklist that follows may be helpful if you are looking to build skills in self-care and de-escalation when your emotional reactions feel outsized or out of control.

For the chart you created in the previous activity "Tracking and De-Escalating Your Trauma Response," you may have asked yourself:

>> What are some strategies I can use for de-escalation during difficult moments?

Many survivors have found the following list of strategies to be helpful for de-escalating an activation response of fight, flight, freeze, or fawn:

>> Breathe. Inhale deeply for a count of three and exhale slowly to a count of five.

>> Tell your partner(s) when you're activated or triggered.

>> Talk to your partner(s) about your specific responses. Let them know what your distress looks like and how they can support you.

>> Report on the feelings rather than act from them: "I can feel my anger rising up; I need a break." Instead of "I can't believe you just said that!"

>> Decide not to argue or shame and blame others when you can feel that you're activated. Practice maintaining this as a boundary.

>> Have one or two close friends you can call for support when your feelings are escalating.

Ground yourself in the present by doing the following:

>> Take your partner's hand, if you can.

>> Make a cup of tea.

>> Literally put your feet on the ground and note where you are.

>> Look around the room at your favorite things or colors.

>> Call a time-out.

>> Take a walk in nature.

The next time you are activated or in a critical moment, use any of the following suggestions to find resources for more support:

>> Build your survivor community.

>> Look for therapeutic help.

>> Consider online and in-person free support groups.

>> Find joyful things to join or attend, like:

- A pottery class

- Sports fan meetups

- Live music events

- Plays or dance performances

>> Identify alternative therapies, such as:

- Acupuncture

- Herbal medicine

- Bodywork or massage

- Sports teams or dance classes

- Swimming or walking

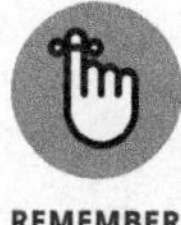

REMEMBER

If you work at it, and have a lot of great support, you can identify your triggers and develop your own strategies and resources for de-escalation. As you grow awareness and heal, kink play can create multiple opportunities for self-reflection and growth. In Appendix B, you can find books and organizations that offer helpful resources as you undertake this life-changing work.

Acknowledging to yourself that you have a history of childhood or adult trauma can be difficult. The narrative you have created around your childhood is often a foundation for how you move in the world — how you introduce yourself and how you talk about yourself to colleagues and friends. Even if that trauma doesn't seem so present in your day-to-day life, the stories you've told yourself about how you grew up, or about your first love, or your college experiences are like a river flowing through you, part of your life force. Re-considering them with an eye on harm and abuse can create monumental shifts in how you see yourself and who you keep close.

Many people have survived traumatic events that were beyond their control. Very often, the situation or events were denied, so their story was buried. If that's true for you, it's likely you didn't get appropriate care for years, or maybe ever. And all of this may have added up over time, making your adult intimate relationships fraught or difficult to navigate.

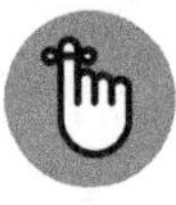

But this doesn't have to be the end of your story. After you accept your trauma history and start to take a look at how it's operating in your adult relationships, you have options. You can start to heal and grow. You can identify the strengths that surviving trauma has forged in your adult coping strategies and also let go of what isn't working.

SURVIVOR SUPER SENSES. This exercise helps you appreciate your strengths as a trauma survivor. It may be easy for you to enumerate the hardships you've endured and the "problematic" coping strategies you've developed. But surviving abuse or a crisis situation as a child or adult also leaves you with gifts that can be difficult to recognize or easy to dismiss. If you're not sure what that means for you, take a minute with this checklist of common strengths that Jaime has noted about herself as a survivor:

>> I have great intuition and can often sense impending trouble or argument.

>> I can tell when people are lying.

>> I'm an excellent de-escalator of other people's activation.

>> I'm a great crisis manager.

>> I can walk into any gathering and read the room — I have hyper-perception of people and situations.

>> Because I dissociate, I can endure boring or uncomfortable situations — like a terrible staff meeting — better than most of my peers.

>> I'm good at distracting people from their distress because when my parents argued when I was young, I did this with my siblings.

>> I can endure tough times.

>> I show up for my friends.

As you start to consider whether kink play or relationships are right for you, remember to take in your strengths as well as your challenges.

For example, Jaime once had a client who went into treatment for alcoholism and an entire team of psychiatrists and physicians gathered to talk about her family history of neglect and abuse. The client was outraged. Her parents had done the best they could with a terrible set of circumstances. She rejected their diagnosis of depression. And when she left rehab, she returned to work with Jaime on her persistently absent libido.

They had a very challenging series of conversations over many months that eventually boiled down to two key insights:

>> In terrible circumstances, your parents can work monumentally hard to provide for you, and you can still be left traumatized by what you were exposed to and what you didn't get around safety and comfort.

>> The things you can see in your adult landscape are breadcrumbs that lead back to a formative history of trauma. In this client's case, she had several issues: alcoholism, a despairingly low libido, consistent sadness that made it hard to get out of bed and go to work, a lot of ruptures in her friendships and family relationships, as well as a number of exes who were mean or abusive.

If this chapter is helping you identify and accept your own trauma history, you may want to do the exercises in Chapter 7 to get a sense what kind of healing work to pursue so that you can live your best kinky life. For some, this might mean starting to chart the impacts of trauma on your relationships. For others, it might mean joining a survivor's group.

As you start to consider whether kink play or relationships are right for you, don't forget to examine your strengths as well as your challenges.

Drawing on Kink as a Way to Heal

You can find endless articles about how psychologically taxing or even dangerous kink is, or how painful it can be for survivors to navigate jealousy in sexually experimental contexts or communities. But not nearly enough ink has been dedicated to exploring the healing possibilities embedded in kink, especially for trauma survivors. In the following sections, you can read about survivors who have made leaps in their healing processes and how they address their trauma triggers through kinky practices and partnerships. With this information, you can begin to consider whether kink might present healing possibilities for you, too.

Liberating kink conversations

Many core kink values and practices — like co-creating consent and building scene containers, centering your pleasure, and talking with friends and lovers about your unrealized desires — pose a tremendous counterpoint to childhood experiences of trauma. They're literally the opposite of abuse, which thrives on secrecy, denial, abuses of power, and contempt.

Trauma survivors who explore kink can find it tremendously liberating to openly discuss things like desire, sexual practices, intimacy, jealousy, insecurity, bodily autonomy, ecstatic psychological states, and lust with multiple scene partners. Consider Ignacio's story, for example:

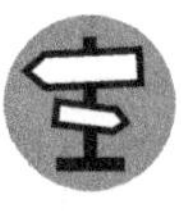

I was always very invested in the negotiation part, the communication part. Let's talk about it all, let's put it out on the table. Let's talk about what we want, what we don't want, what's good, and what's bad because in my family of origin, I never got to have that agency or any kind of communication whatsoever to shape my reality. None at all. It was just given to me — imposed — and I had to accept it with physical punishment, emotional punishment, and my sister's sexual abuse. So that's where kink discussions really became a healing practice for me.
—Ignacio

Using coping strategies

Here are some strategies survivors draw on — sometimes purposefully, some-times involuntarily — to cope with activation. Knowing when your coping strategies are operating can greatly improve your relationship to them, and their usefulness.

>> **Dissociation.** For a lot of survivors, dissociation becomes a go-to tool for survival. *Dissociation* means that when you're in crisis, you can remove yourself emotionally from the present. Your body can show up, but your mind and your spirit are safely elsewhere.

Some survivors appear to be *spacing out* while they dissociate or perhaps they observe themselves from across the room. Other people develop alternative personas while dissociating, a proxy or surrogate personality to help get through difficult challenges.

Note: Euphoric dissociation is induced consensually (discussed in Chapter 10) and can lead to bliss. Dissociative coping is induced by a crisis or threatening event, and is often a means of self-protection.

>> **Compartmentalization.** If you're managing a lot of responsibilities or find yourself highly activated with your kink scene partner because intimacy can be challenging, *compartmentalization* allows you to file or lock away one set of experiences while you attend to another.

Survivors often compartmentalize traumatic memories so that they can work with them at a reasonable pace and live their lives. Kink survivors may compartmentalize challenging situations in order to de-escalate fear-based responses and attend to the person or the moment at hand.

» **Splitting.** When you engage in *splitting*, you can assign qualities to one person or another to help you cope with your fear in the moment, for instance: Mom/ good, Dad/bad; Me/good, ex-lover/bad; and friend/good, crush/bad. When you were in actual jeopardy, splitting probably helped you identify a supporter who could get you through a terrifying moment. But in the real world, and in your adult relationships, the truth is usually much more complex.

Part of your healing work is to embrace and manage a much more integrated, complex reality, such as: Mom/overwhelmed, Dad/absent; Me/struggling and shut down, ex-lover struggling and volatile; and friend/wonderful and comforting, crush/wonderful but scary because I have too many feelings.

As you begin to heal, you can start to recognize when you're using these coping strategies to fragment yourself or simplify the situation as a protective measure. With this knowledge, you can make choices about whether or when to use them, which is called *integration*.

It's not always wise to be fully integrated in the moment, depending on how intensely a current situation mimics past abuse or triggers a traumatic response. However, the great thing about healing is that as you become more aware of your coping strategies, you can decide what to do rather than find yourself at the mercy of an involuntary reaction.

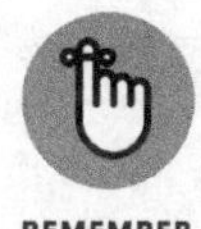

As a survivor, you are likely already adept at moving through various kinds of altered states to manage your daily life and intimate connections. The altered emotional states that your kink activities bring you to can create a tender bridge to your survivor-self. In any given scene, you may encounter your memories, your coping personas, and feelings you keep deeply buried to protect yourself. Many survivor-kinksters find new possibilities in these encounters for healing, loosening their burdens, and letting go.

Trying on new parts of yourself with different partners

Any time you enter into a relationship with a new playmate or lover, you enter into a new realm of possibility. You put yourself in the path of someone else's worldview, ways of being, and circles of loved ones and passion. Your world gets bigger and often reorients itself as you attempt to accommodate the wildness and wonder of being intimate with this new person.

In kink relationships and social worlds, the reach and intensity of love and play can extend outward into groups of intersecting or parallel circles. This expansiveness has special significance for trauma survivors, especially if you've compartmentalized parts of your trauma history as a way of managing it. As you heal, survivors can spend a lot of time compartmentalizing experiences and carefully re-integrating them on the path to wellness. In many ways, kink relational practices create very similar pathways as you create different levels of emotional investment in your kink play and manage a complex intimate life.

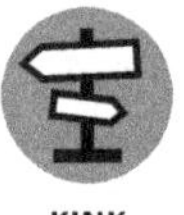

The way that I tried to rework my emotional and sexual trauma in my kink world was through family re-creations. Role-play and family re-creations — that was huge for me and my healing. Before I even had language for it, I was re-creating my family dynamic, over and over in all kinds of relationships. I was trying to fix the lack of communication, the lack of connection, and the fear. I found myself constantly re-creating scenarios. My brother had been my protector in my childhood, and my sister was my abuser. So through kink role-play, I'd create a brother and a sister and put everyone into specific roles when I played with them. I'd re-create all kinds of scenes that hurt me, but here among people who love me, I could create better ways for these things to occur that are pleasurable and joy-producing, rather than the fear and secrecy and pain. **—Ignacio**

Here, Ignacio recognizes that both their polyamorous constellation (their expansive mix of lovers and partners) and their kink practices helped them role-play toxic family dynamics and transform them into new, healing experiences.

This is a common strategy for many survivors, and one that has often been stigmatized or judged. How can you heal if you're drawing on abusive stories in your intimacy, sexuality, or play? The answer is simple: In abusive situations, your choices are stolen from you, as Ignacio notes. In your chosen kinky families, you're the author of your stories. You can create what you want. You can criticize without repercussions. You can play with consensual pain, terrorism, or hitting without harming anyone. You're free to leave. Many survivors draw on the multiple, intimate bonds they create and the intensity of kink play to rework and transform painful family-of-origin stories.

Transforming your story

There are numerous critiques of kink scenarios being used to rework past trauma. Many people find this kind of intimate re-creation and exploration terrifying, and therefore designate any such play as fundamentally toxic. But survivor testimonies over the past few decades have soundly refuted this analysis.

Of course, re-creation and role-play that parallels or mimics your abuse is risky. So is dating. So is falling in love.

Do you trust your partners? Do they respect you deeply? Do they honor your journey as a survivor? If so, they may be candidates for this kind of connection.

Or not. Only you know what is transformative in your journey toward meaningful intimacy. Only you are the expert on your healing. A good litmus test about the value or efficacy of this kind of play is to simply review how it's impacting your life. Ask yourself:

>> Are you falling into depression? Or are you uplifted and experiencing deeper joy?

>> Is trust and love growing in your kinky social and intimate life? Or are your limits being ignored and has conflict become a constant?

>> Can you take care of your basic responsibilities — getting to work, paying your bills, parenting? Is your life unraveling, or are you unable to take care of your life as you did before?

>> Can you take care of yourself? Or is your basic ability to get out of bed in the morning, face your day, groom yourself, and attend to your friendships?

Transforming your trauma through role-play and other re-creation scenarios can make life better, more spacious and more joyful if you have a strong healing foundation and if you have chosen worthy scene partners. If the opposite is true, and this kind of intimacy and play is creating pain and chaos in your life, then it's time to take a break and get more support for your healing process.

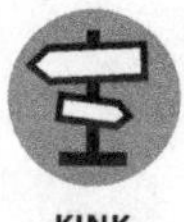

KINK STORY

A paradox for me as a survivor was when I engaged in a rape-play fantasy, where I assumed the role of aggressor. The scene was meticulously negotiated, filled with raw intensity — struggle, aggression, and primal physicality. Every muscle engaged, every sensation heightened, it was visceral and empowering. Afterward, I felt like a primal force, my body pulsating with energy and awareness. It was a transformative moment where boundaries were explored and desires met in a safe, consensual space. —**Ignacio**

Honoring Your Story

You may have spent a lot of your life burying the story of your childhood or adult trauma. It may have taken you many years to recognize that what happened was real or wrong. That's true for so many people.

Coming to honor your story, to uncover and know what you know, may be difficult. You can acknowledge it, and in doing so, you stand with your survivor self. What does this even mean? The following sections explore what it means to grow respect for your survivor story and keep faith with yourself.

Honoring your limits is a strength

Continually feeling yourself at the edge of your limits around emotional capacity, flexibility, and intimacy is difficult. As a trauma survivor, you may want to make everything be okay for everyone else. You may be tired of having to speak up and say what's really happening for you, especially if your lover or scene partner is excited about a new kink or intimate practice that they have proposed. You may wonder: why do I always have to be the one to set limits or introduce a concern?

But the truth is, people who care about you want to know and respect your limits. They want to know *you.* As you move through your healing journey and become truly intimate with others, you'll find it easier and easier to speak your truth among your loved ones and:

>> Know when to stop or tap out.

>> Understand that it's okay to be overwhelmed.

>> Tell anyone, and especially yourself, when you need to: "I can't do this."

>> Know that it's okay to be done trying.

REMEMBER

It's okay to be honest with your scene partners or lovers. You are responsible for setting limits that take care of you; and in the end, take very good care of your partners as well.

It's not your job to:

>> Heal others.

>> Please others at your expense.

>> Make it work if the effort isn't mutual.

>> Constantly compromise, without reciprocity.

>> Anticipate others' needs.

>> Change yourself to fit in.

It *is* your job to:

>> Heal — as much as you possibly can.

>> Listen to yourself — to your needs and desires.

>> Respect yourself and your time.

>> Be honest with and true to yourself.

>> Protect your energy by setting limits.

» Leave when you're not being valued.

» Say *No* when you need to and Say *Yes* when it's good for you.

Taking care of yourself, in community

You can use *pod mapping,* a tool created by Mia Mingus and the Bay Area Transformative Justice Collective (BATJC) to help assess your support system as you consider exploring and experimenting with kink.

Designed to help BATJC members get through times of crisis by diagramming a pod of supporters, the handy map became a go-to resource for people experiencing health or family crises or those trying to escape violent situations.

We've adapted this tool (see Figure 11-1) and used it for many years to assess whether we have the right balance of close friends and socializing, daily love connections, trained health professionals, and joy spaces in our lives. Our pod maps create the core scaffolding of our health and vitality. It's made all of our kinky exploration possible. When we experience big changes, and people drop off the map, we know we need to recruit someone new into the mix or build in a new practice to shore us up.

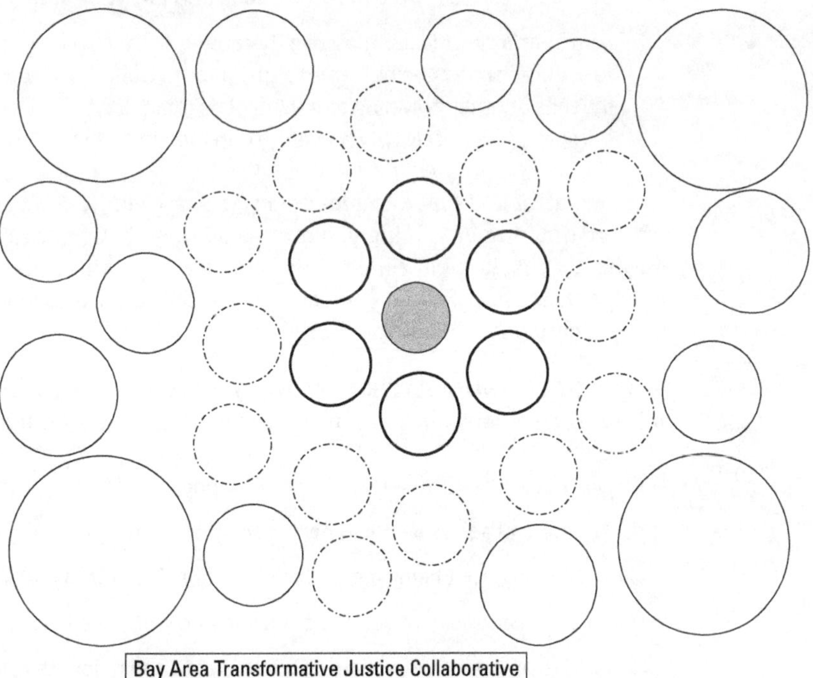

FIGURE 11-1:
My pod map.

Pod mapping can help you look closely at your community of friends and confidantes as you consider and pursue kink relationships. Do you have a lot of support? Is your pod full of highly judgmental, anti-kink people? Mapping your pod can help you see what kind of community-building you need to do to create an environment where you can explore kink with joy and expansiveness.

To create your own pod map, follow these steps:

1. **Place yourself at the center of your pod map.**

2. **Fill in the names of people you trust the most in the six dark-lined circles around you.**

   These are the people you can count on to be in your corner, no matter what. You may not have six people, and the map helps you think about whether you need more confidantes and supporters to grow your kink life.

3. **Add the names of other people you rely on in the dotted circles.**

   The dotted circles represent people who know you less intimately than your group of six, but they bring fun, energy, support, and laughter to your days. Your crushes or scene partners may be in the dotted circles. Wonderful people you see only a few times a year or colleagues whose work really supports you may be dotted-circle people.

4. **On the outside, in the larger circles, pencil in professionals, resources, or practices that you can rely on to round out your life.**

   Jaime has a spectacular massage therapist and life coach in one of her big four outer circles; seeing her favorite bands on tour as much as possible inhabits another; traveling to Ireland periodically to visit her cousins is in a third; and her weekly NA recovery group meeting is in the fourth circle.

If you create a pod that has a lot of empty spaces in it, or a pod filled with people who are draining or judging you every day, then that's good information to have. Maybe it's not the right time to take a big leap into kinky play. Maybe it's time to build your support pod so you can start to find kinksters who share your values and are passionate about the things you care about.

ACTIVITY

WHO'S HERE AND WHAT'S MISSING? As a survivor of trauma, ask yourself the following questions on your journey to building a pod that fully supports you:

» Do I have other trauma survivors in my pod?

» Are there other survivors in my growing kink network?

» Am I open about being a survivor among people I play with? Why/not?

» Is conversation about survivors hushed and whispered in my community?

» Is there an open conversation about healing and resources and growth?

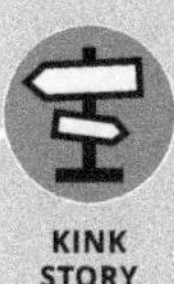

MY FRIENDS MAKE MY KINK WORLD WORK

I grew up in Iran and moved here at 18, and later one of my childhood friends moved here. When I started taking him to kink things in our 20s, he was a novice and was curious. But I could see a lot of things made him uncomfortable. Then over the years, he did a ton of experimentation. And when we saw each other again, it was like our positions had flipped; he has much more kink experience than I do. It has been just incredible to have another person who grew up in my cultural context and is my age — to interpret kink scenes and kink ideas in the U.S. Even my identity as a trauma survivor — coming from Iran, we have a really different framework and experience of violence and various systems of power than our friends who grew up here. Being with him and talking about what's going on in our lives and in our kinky fantasies and scenes, he's really the only one in my life who can share all of these things on such a deep and formative level. It's a singular bond that contextualizes my experiences as a survivor and makes my kink life so much richer. **—Aredvi**

Living in a community where there's open, engaging conversation on survivorship is an unparalleled, foundational support in any survivor's healing process. When you can freely share your resources, experiences of growth, mistakes, funny stories, failures, and major milestones in recovery, then life is fuller and possibilities abound.

Keeping the faith

When you're struggling to understand your survivor story and how your traumatic history is impacting your relationships, you can easily lose faith in yourself. The daily climb toward wellness can seem insurmountable at times. You can become exhausted and think: *I'm just going to stop having relationships altogether. I'm fine on my own. I can't do this.*

But you can do this. You can grow. If kink expression and connection is what you want in your adult relationships, you deserve the space to explore and discover these possibilities just as much as anyone else. You can keep faith with your survivor self by believing in your ability to do your best to learn and to keep trying. You deserve a life full of the best love you can give and the most bountiful love you can accept.

Chapter **12**

Working Out Struggles in Kink Relationships

Everyone struggles in relationships. BFFs struggle with their limited free time and various priorities. Monogamous couples wrestle with the demands of emotional and sexual exclusivity. Kinky single people labor to find good scene partners and community. Polyamorous people with differing needs around intimacy and kink struggle to support each other and adapt.

If you are deciding whether to try out kink in your relationship, or to embark upon new kink practices, you might be struggling too.

In this chapter, you can find a lot of support for a few key kink wrestles:

» How can you move from "vanilla" to kinky in your existing relationship?

» How do you deal with desires that don't match your partner's around kink and intimacy?

» How do you manage jealousy in the kink context?

>> Can a breach of trust be repaired? How?

>> How do you know when your relationship has moved away from everyday struggles into toxic or dangerous territory, and what can you do?

Struggle in relationships is universal, and yet struggles in kink relationships are also specific because kink often engages and exposes your most vulnerable self. Therefore, it's important to take extra good care of yourself and your partners as you make your kinky way and build the skills you need to flourish.

Asking Yourself *Why Now*

A best first step in figuring out whether or how to introduce kink into your relationship is getting settled on the why of your exploration. Each person in the partnership should undertake this exercise privately. After you each complete the activity, you can decide whether to share your answers. The important thing is to focus on yourself and to answer the questions as though you'll never share them.

ACTIVITY

ALIVENESS INVENTORY. Give yourself some privacy so you can tune out any competing influences or concerns, like the needs of your partners, parents, or friends. Answer the following questions:

>> What are the ways you're most alive in your partnership right now? What parts of you and your dreams and passions are best supported here?

>> What parts of you are hidden or suppressed — sexually, socially, professionally, artistically, emotionally, and so on?

>> When did you give up or start hiding these parts of you?

>> When you think specifically about your intimate or sexual life in your partnership, how are you most alive and true to yourself?

>> What are your favorite and most satisfying ways of being sexual and/or intimate with your partner or lover?

>> When you think about your sexuality in your partnership, how are you hiding? What have you suppressed out of fear of judgment or fear of scaring off or repulsing your partner?

>> What haven't you said to your partner that really needs saying if you're going to explore your authentic sexuality and consider kink with integrity and care?

>> On a scale of 1 to 10, with 10 being the most extreme, how frustrated or depressed are you by the sacrifices you've made in abandoning or suppressing parts of yourself?

>> On a scale of 1 to 10, with 10 being the most likely, how likely is it that you'll leave or need to break up if you *don't* explore kink in this relationship or in some area of your life?

>> On a scale of 1 to 10, how likely is it that you or your partner will leave or break up if you *do* explore kink in or adjacent to the relationship?

>> What do you think exploring kink will bring into the relationship or solve?

TIP

This reflection exercise is full of emotionally taxing questions, so take your time. The key is to get honest, even if it takes months to complete and share your answers. You can start and stop and come back. Let your answers give you clues about what your next right step might be.

TIP

Some couples may feel confident that they have the tools to be vulnerable and share important truths that their partner may not know, so they can work through these issues together. But if you and your partner finish this exercise and find yourselves struggling with the results, it may be time to get professional help (like a therapist) in order to share each other's thoughts in a supportive environment.

WE REALLY HATE THE V TERM

We *generally* don't use the V term — vanilla — in discussing kinky and non-kinky relationships. One reason is that it equates vanilla with blandness and if you are a baker, you know that's just wrong because vanilla is really the secret sauce.

But a more important reason is that there's a bit of judgment in the construction; it promotes the idea that people who are not kinky are bland or that their sexuality somehow lacks flavor. As a team that has worked with thousands of people all over the world on desire mapping (see Appendix A) — we strenuously object.

All kinds of people who do not engage in kink have wildly interesting and satisfying sexualities and intimate lives. In fact, all kinds of people who do not engage in sex at all have wildly interesting sexualities and intimate lives.

Let's support each other's infinite, and infinitely interesting sexual and intimate practices and expressions — kinky or not.

Managing Asymmetrical Needs Around Kink

Probably the most common request that Jaime gets as a sex coach is to help couples with *asymmetrical* intimacy needs. For example, one partner's libido is significantly more turbo-charged than the other's. Or, one person wants an open relationship, while the other wants to stay monogamous. The asymmetry that we discuss in this section is when one person is interested in kink and the other isn't.

The fact that you and your partner aren't a perfectly matched set around each other's desires or relationship preferences makes sense. Very few couples align on everything that matters to them. Couples who stay happy and connected over the long haul are often:

>> Aligned around core things that matter *the most* to them — things that may or may not be about desire. They could pertain to things like parenting, politics, or the flow of your social and daily lives.

>> Able to adapt or be flexible about core needs their partner has that are outside of their interests or comfort zones. Sometimes this pertains to being open about how differently a partner pursues their desire. But often, these divergent interests are centered on things like traveling, spending lots of time with friends or family, or having an ambition or passion that demands a lot of focus or energy.

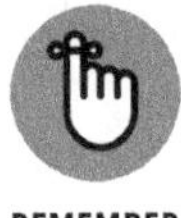

REMEMBER

Being in relationship means being in a constant state of compromise. Despite all the rom-com hype about finding a perfect soulmate or "the one," very few people in long-term partnerships find themselves in a situation where they don't have to give up on some significant wants in order to stay together.

The challenges that couples with differing needs around kink may include:

>> You may feel frightened or repulsed by the kink your partner is interested in.

>> You may be in a sexually-exclusive relationship and exploring kink may veer into new territories — with others.

>> While you may be interested in whatever kink your partner has described, you may have no skills or expertise in that arena and worry how you will be able to meet that need.

>> This topic may feel beyond what you committed to when you got together, or even at odds with your values or religious practices.

This might seem like a daunting array of barriers, even if only one of them is on your list. But many of Jaime's clients who work through their challenges have been able to enjoy significant benefits in their relationship via kink exploration. So likewise, you may be able to:

>> Experience or stretch into parts of yourself that have been hidden or buried in your relationship.

>> Find (mutually affirmed) partners or additional lovers who enjoy things your partner hates or can't be a part of.

>> Acquire new skills and kink practices that you feel proud of.

>> Engage in new conversation and grow new friendships around your kinky wants and needs.

>> Drop resentments and stop having the same old fight with your partner over the things that you can't get from them.

By adding these new pleasures and possibilities into the mix, you could bring a lighter, renewed, or more joyful self to your relationship with your partner.

All of these exciting changes are possible when opening up to kink possibilities, but they're certainly not a given or a guarantee. Exploring kink with care, transparency, and full consent is critical to the success of the endeavor. Mallory recounts in the following Kink Story how she and her partner managed asymmetry in a way that in the end, brought them more pleasure.

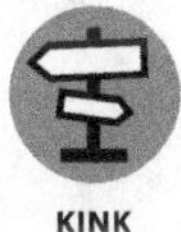

KINK STORY

My gal pal and I encountered an interesting conundrum in our play: I like to engage in playful and even bratty talk when bottoming during a scene, while she likes not having to talk and being able to just sink into Topspace. After a few awkward attempts where our play just didn't quite land right for either of us, we decided to bring this asymmetry into the center of our play! We negotiated a predicament for our scenes: my role was to keep talking and her role was to make me stop talking, and I would be punished further if I kept talking. This created a fun and delightful tension that worked perfectly for us. —**Mallory.**

Operating with Intention

If you are ready to address asymmetrical desires in your partnership, you'll want to take great care of each other. Because once you have opened the conversation about kink possibilities, differences in your desires that may have been entirely invisible become clear. You may have fantasized about light bondage, while your partner is interested in sadism. You may be developing an identity as a Furry and your partner is not interested in role-play of any kind (see Chapter 4 for more on kink likes and practices).

Revealing these differences can feel scary, like you've found deal-breakers that you didn't know existed. But the important thing to do during this period of time is to:

1. Put everything on the table.

2. Breathe. You don't have to solve everything in this minute.

3. Let these truths rest on you, take yourself and your partner in.

The sections that follow outline three key guiding principles to support you during the discovery process.

Exploring with care

Exploring *with care* means:

>> You co-create agreements at the start — rather than, say, come home from a work trip and tell your partner you went to a sex club.

>> You make sure *each of you* are pursuing desires that matter to you and align with your values.

>> You don't run off with a new crush or disappear into a kink social group.

>> You keep your agreements (see Chapter 8 for more information on creating agreements.)

Being transparent

Transparency means very simply: *no secrets.*

>> You aren't hiding a crush or a hidden agenda as you create agreements.

>> You aren't agreeing to boundaries you know you'll violate because you just want to get to a "yes" from your partner on kink exploration.

>> If you can't be honest in opening discussions about kink, it's unlikely that you're going to be able to be honest when you actually try to make new agreements or try out kink practices.

>> If you are afraid that your partner will harm you if you tell them about your kinky fantasies or desires, get help. *Safety first.*

Committing to full consent

Here's what *full consent* means:

>> Sharing as much as possible about yourself and what your desires, intentions, and hopes are.

>> Listening deeply to what your partner is telling you about their needs and desires.

>> Rejecting coercive control. No one person in the relationship is held hostage to a relationship demand, such as a partner's housing being at risk because they didn't agree to experiment with kink.

FUNDAMENTALS: I'M VANILLA (OR KINKY) IT'S JUST WHO I AM

I often work with couples who have *asymmetrical needs* around their intimacy — that is, one person states that they're wholly vanilla and the other reports that they are fundamentally kinky.

My question for partners who present this asymmetry as a fundamental dilemma is:

Is it more important for you to live out this part of you — this *fundamental way of relating* — or is it more important for you to stay with your partner?

My clients hate this question. It often feels impossible to answer because it's so starkly either/or, but that's the nature of fundamentals. If this relational way of being is indeed essential to you, and the opposite is essential to your partner, then you have no need for a second coaching session. You have to decide between these two things.

Because if it's more important for you to stay with your partner, then your vanilla or kink intimacy needs aren't quite fundamental. In other words, if you can modify your ideas or practices around this deeply held way of being and have some wiggle room to discover, flow, or ratchet back your fundamental identity or needs — then there's often a third way to explore, and a possible way forward together. **—Jaime**

Investigating a Third Way

Most of the couples and polycules that Jaime works with have divergent kinky desires. Some discover that they are both Dominants or both submissives. Others find that their partner's interests are way beyond anything they want be a part of or even know about. Many couples fall into less polarized territories — their partners are interested in things they haven't considered or aren't unfamiliar with.

In all of these cases, the work is to try to seek *a third way* together. This is especially true for partners who are aligned on their shared values and whose relationships have built the kind of joy, community, and family that meets their core needs. Differences around kinky desires do not have to be a deal-breaker. There are a lot of ways to move forward beyond either-or thinking about kink in your life.

Are you ready to work toward a third way? If your relationship is grounded, your third-way exploration is going to be more productive. If not, you'll have a harder time and need more support to process what's happening for you and in your relationship. The following exercise can shed some light on how you and your partner can proceed.

ACTIVITY

THIRD-WAY INVESTIGATION. For this exercise, ask yourselves the questions that follow:

Question 1: What could be a fun, low-stakes beginning activity to start to try kink out? Pick things that you could suggest to your partner, for example:

>> Trying out kink fetishwear at home.

>> Engaging in an activity you've been fantasizing about. Start with something small that feels doable to both of you.

>> Crafting hypothetical kink profiles together, without posting them. The process of describing yourselves can be fun and revealing.

>> Cruising together at a kinky event — identifying activities that look interesting or turn you on. Let each other know which roles interest you and who you would want to be in the scenario.

>> Defining an ideal first exploration together and figuring out how to pursue this ideal.

>> Defining separate first explorations together and figuring out how to support each other pursing these separately.

>> If one or both of you wants to know very little about each other's exploration, helping to create a structure that supports each other's privacy, and your ability to manage this new kink space in your relationship.

Question 2: What could you let go of in terms of your need to either control or accelerate this process that would take great care of your partner?

>> Creating a series of compromise scenarios that addresses your bottom-line needs and meets some of theirs.

>> Initiating fun and playful discussion about possible kink exploration, moving away from the continual arguments you've been in.

>> Initiating a dinner with kinky friends or another couple that is in exploring kink to either get support or cruise them.

Question 3: Do we both need to try out kink?

>> Understanding that having asymmetrical needs sometimes means that one person needs a kink play partner or play space and the other needs deeper intimacy with their friends or needs more childcare so they have time to themselves or is able to finally make music or get an art studio.

>> Choosing a kinky third-way solution can be extremely relieving and exciting, while often drawing skepticism from people outside of your relationship. So be careful when choosing confidantes as you are likely to be tender while you experiment.

>> The point is to meet both of your core needs, not to do the same thing. What others think doesn't matter. What matters is what the two of you think.

TIP

When you're creating third-way options, be generous with your partner. You may find yourself holding more power in the moment, but that may not always be true across the long span of your relationship. Many people come to regret their failure to own and mediate the impacts of their power after it has shifted in their relationship over time.

Finding a third way is an exercise in sharing power, so that everyone gets their fair share of the goodies — even if the content differs considerably.

REMEMBER

Our favorite way to think about third way ideas is to keep it HOT:

>> **H:** Honor where you are at as a couple or team.

>> **O:** Offer something to your partner to counter polarized thinking. What's possible? What could work?

>> **T:** Try something. Break the stalemate.

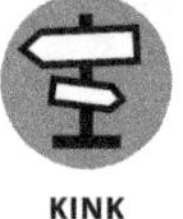

I'm a Top, and my wife is a Top-heavy switch (see Appendix A). She loves bondage as a bottom, and I am not into bondage at all. Our solution? She can bottom to a rope Top whenever she wants to because we negotiated for our wants, needs, desires years ago. And we keep the lines of communication open all the time in case something changes or comes up. It's also because we trust each other when we play with others. This has really worked out well for us. —**Naria**

Taking a Communications Inventory

If you are frustrated as a communicator in your relationships, your tendency might be to focus on your partners and everything they are or are not doing and giving. But great communication starts with you. In this section, you can start to think about yourself as a communicator in your relationship and whether you need to build more awareness or tools to "fight fairly" or navigate painful territory.

Communicating your desires

If you aren't sure whether you and your partner are capable of discussing your kink fantasies or desires in a way that shows mutual respect and care, taking a communications inventory may help you. Are you a constructive communicator? Do you shame and blame your partner in the heat of arguments? The following exercise may help you gain a sense of your and your partner's capacity for taking on emotionally taxing conversations.

COMMUNICATIONS INVENTORY. As you prepare to share with a partner the kink desires that you may have identified through the activities in Chapters 4 and 5, the following inventory can help you evaluate your readiness as affirming communicators. Take your time and score your relationship here:

>> **Communicating constructively:** Score 1 to 5 with 1 being that you experience repeating, fraught, and unresolved conflicts and 5 being that you are excellent at getting to resolution. Ask yourself:

- What is conflict like between us?

- Do we resolve differences reasonably?

- Are our conflicts cyclical, intense, and never ending?

>> **Fighting fairly:** Determine whether you can resolve conflict without shaming, blaming, shouting at, or hurting each other. Score 1 to 5 with 1 being you or your partner (at times or often) inflict serious emotional or even physical harm

and 5 being that no one resorts to any (or almost none) of the listed harmful fighting behaviors.

>> **Owning your part:** Score 1 to 5 with 1 if one or both of you believes that you *never have a part* in the difficulty; it's all on the other person. And 5 for if both of you are largely self-referencing when you have arguments.

- Can each person take responsibility for their contribution to the current conflict? That earns a 5 score.

- Can you see and own what part you are playing in the difficulty? If It's only you, that earns a 3.

>> **Staying cool:** Determine whether you can stay kind and supportive to each other even when you're angry or upset. Score 1 to 5 with 1 being you both absolutely can't do this; and 5 being you're both able to be reasonably supportive even when upset.

>> **Finding support:** Assess whether you have good people to confide in about the relationship who don't trash your partner or have an agenda for the relationship. Score 1 to 5 with 1 being neither of you have anyone like this and 5 being you both do.

If you find your score to be in the 5 to 12 range — we suggest taking classes, getting counseling, and/or finding resources on building accountable, nonviolent communication strategies (refer to Appendix A on accountability).

Tolerating not knowing

Couples who do well in opening up their relationships to kink are good at managing their feelings when they don't know what's coming next. Some couples manage to adapt to lots of changes over the course of their relationship — deaths in the family, being fired from jobs, having children, moving out of state, or out of the country. These fast adapters are well-suited to trying out kink. Because the reality is, like all of us in any relationship, *you really don't know what's coming next.*

Do expect the unexpected

You can plan all the plans you want together, but you can't control outcomes. You may have very clear ideas about how trying out kink will go for you, what you're capable of, and where your limits are. But a year from now, all your ideas may be obsolete. The actual experience of opening up to new intimacies and new parts of yourself, while your partner does the same, isn't entirely predictable.

Don't catastrophize

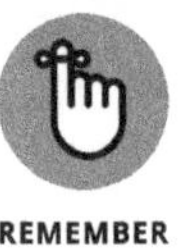

REMEMBER

If all goes well, some wonderful things will happen. You may discover some new intimate ways of relating that open up your world, bring immeasurable joy, and strengthen your relationship. Undoubtedly, though, mistakes will be made. Miscommunication, hurts, and missteps will happen. That's okay. You're human. So's your partner. Take responsibility, apologize, work it out, and keep going. You're in this together.

Owning and Rejecting Jealousy

When opening an existing relationship to kink, the potential for jealous reactivity is high. Often, kink exploration involves observing others engaging in kinky play. If you've never watched other couples or groups connect intimately, this can be a huge leap for you and your partner. Sometimes kink discovery involves joining a new social group or taking classes to build skills. These activities introduce you to a world of novice and experienced kinksters who like you — are fun, curious, attractive people. And for many, kink experimentation involves inviting other kinksters into your intimate lives through play.

You and your partner may feel overwhelmed by the brilliance and creativity of the kinksters you encounter. If you feel insecure about your relationship or embarrassed about being a kink novice, you may find yourself jealous or self-deprecating and need support. In this section, you can find great tools for dealing with envy and jealousy as you step into kink community.

Realizing that jealousy is a scarcity response

Today's culture projects and generates *scarcity* (a world of diminishing resources and opportunities) at every corner. Capitalism as an organizing structure literally runs on scarcity and competition. Even as a child, your life was steeped in competitive contests — from your sports teams to your grades in elementary school. Nearly everyone is formed inside a system that tells you that competition is good, and if you want to have a good life, you must compete to land at the top of the heap.

Jealousy then, is a crucial part of this system. If only one (country, scholar, lover) can be the best, the smartest, and the worthiest, then all the others are losers. The consequences can seem overwhelming — from not getting into that top college, to failing to obtain that dream job, to living a penniless, lonely life.

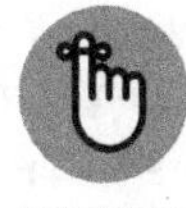

REMEMBER

Jealousy is your internal alarm system to detect threats against the lover you must acquire to win the ultimate-partner game. Accordingly, people grow into their romantic and intimate lives fueled with anxiety about not being enough, and ultimately, losing and being left behind.

ACTIVITY

WHAT WOULD IT MEAN TO BE ENOUGH? A fundamental viewpoint in a scarcity-driven culture is that you are not enough. You may have internalized this without knowing it. Ask yourself:

>> What is your first memory of feeling like you weren't enough — too big or too small, not smart, cute, funny, strong, or hot enough?

>> In this memory, how old are you? Who is telling you this?

>> What kind of impact did this have?

>> What is your most humiliating memory of being not enough?

>> How do you think this impacts you today?

>> Are the messengers or catalysts in these scenarios trustworthy?

>> Have the messengers in these scenarios harmed you in other ways?

>> How or why are you giving them power?

>> What if you could stop believing these lies?

>> What would life be like in a world where you are enough?

Keep these notes with you as you move through this section on jealousy.

Monogamy culture reinforces jealousy

Monogamy and marriage fit neatly into the overarching competitive system of society because they align to push you to choose one person early in your lifetime, or you'll lose out. All the good partners will be taken if you don't get yourself into a position to be an attractive partner — physically, socially, materially. Time is *so short* to prove that you're the best catch.

Monogamy culture tells you that good people are disappearing every day, and you'll likely end up alone if you don't figure it out now.

Getting out of this mind-set is no small thing. It's scary. Depending on the expectations of your family of origin and your friendship circle, it may be driving a significant percentage of conversation and activity especially while you're in your 20s and 30s.

What would it be like to get off of this competition and scarcity train? What if love were abundant and to be shared? What if you could love your partner and also tolerate that your desires may be different, or that you need to explore them with other people?

While many kinky couples live their kink lives only relating to one another sexually, kink life has an expansive view of play, partnership, sex, and intimacy. Moving into kink spaces means meeting many people who practice non-monogamy (see Appendix A) and are enjoying a spectrum of intimate relationships via their kink play.

It's perfectly fine to maintain a monogamous life in kink society. Many kinksters question all kinds of norms in intimacy. And in doing so, they may push the limits set by monogamy as a standard that champions jealousy as an essential aspect of love.

If you are open to the many ways kinksters organize their intimate lives, you will observe that de-escalating jealous conflicts and rejecting jealousy as an expression of love has the potential to free you from so many emotional and intimate constraints.

Kink culture can stigmatize jealousy

Monogamy culture isn't the only culture that has a problem with jealousy. In kink circles, jealousy can be stigmatized as uncool or immature. The story goes: If you're a true kinkster, you don't experience jealousy, *which is utter nonsense!*

You don't suddenly live outside of this overwhelming monogamy-centric, scarcity culture when you start considering kink. Consider all the envies and jealousies of your upbringing, the excruciating formative romances in your teens, and your early dating history. These experiences combine in your life as you find yourself at this point of curiosity or exploration. Just because you don't *want* to be jealous doesn't mean that you won't be. Aspiring to move beyond jealousy and possessiveness in your dating and partnering life doesn't mean this is where you are today.

Feeling jealous as you explore kinky connections is very common and perfectly okay. Things will go a lot better if you can own and discuss your jealousy with your loved ones, rather than deny it and act out of scarcity-driven fear.

Discovering your jealousy triggers

As you think about how jealousy might be operating as you consider kink experimentation, a constructive step toward addressing or de-escalating your jealousy
is discovering your *triggers* — what sets you off when you feel threatened.

Working on letting go of controlling or possessive thoughts and behaviors starts
with discovering when and under what circumstances you are likely to be *activated*
around your jealousy (see Appendix A for the definition).

ACTIVITY

KNOWING WHEN YOU'RE MOST VULNERABLE. This exercise can help you sift
through the circumstances that leave you most at risk for jealous reactivity.

1. Ask yourself this question: When are you most vulnerable to jealousy?

   - Early on in a relationship?

   - When your partner announces a new crush?

   - When you're overextended at work or as a parent?

   - When you haven't had a vacation in more than a year?

   - When you're getting all the drudgery while your partner has all the fun?

   - When you're not feeling well physically?

   - When your depression is weighing you down?

   - When your partner goes to a kink party without you?

   The possibilities are endless. Dig a little and think about the history of jealous
   blowups in your current and past relationships and how they've ignited. What
   conditions make you more vulnerable to jealousy?

2. List your biggest fights or explosions around jealousy.

   - Look to see if a pattern emerges or any particular trends around your
     vulnerability. Determine whether you can ask your partner to say or do
     something to head off the kind of distress you've encountered previously.

   - If you can, identify what has worked in terms of taking care of yourself
     and your jealousy in the past. What's a tried-and-true method to care for
     yourself during jealous episodes?

The material you've gained from answering these two questions can form a foundation for noticing when you're vulnerable, so you can back away from reactive
jealousy. It can be a guidepost to figuring out how to ask for help and reassurance.

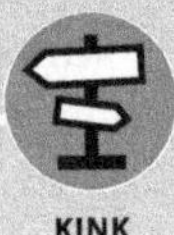

KINK STORY

IF YOU'RE IN YOUR PARTNER'S PHONE, THERE'S NO GOOD NEWS

During one particularly gruesome period of jealousy and obsession with a partner, I started surveilling them. We shared a computer and sometimes they left various private modes of communication open by mistake. They didn't always have a password on their phone. We had an open relationship, but I was certain they were involved in various kinds of relationships that were off limits per our agreements.

This was a truly terrible time in my life. We had moved to a new state, and I had no intimate friends locally. My new employer was abusive. We were in a much less diverse community — our mixed-race, queer family was visibly strange in the environment, drawing unwanted and even hostile attention. The kids were young, and parenting demands were high. Looking back on this time, it makes sense to me that I came to over rely on my partner and to imagine threats to my sense of security.

And what was on their computer or in their phone? It doesn't matter. After you break your partner's trust by invading their privacy, the relationship is mortally wounded. What you may have discovered is beside the point. Unless you're capable of coming clean and making radical changes, this kind of trust breach is very, very hard to come back from. **—Jaime**

WARNING

Jealousy lives inside the terror of scarcity, and it also shrinks possibility at every corner. It *creates scarcity by shutting everyone out.*

Jealousy creates the very thing you would want to avoid in your relationship — a distant, resentful partner, rather than an intimate partner who can hold and soothe you through your most vulnerable moments.

TIP

If you're feeling tortured by jealousy — if it feels constant or nagging or intrusive in your daily life — your mental and physical health may be in jeopardy. If so, seek help (refer to Appendix B for resources).

Creating Support Versus Judgment

Probably the biggest mistake you can make around dealing with jealousy is to ascend to a place of superiority and judgment about how uncool it is for your partner to feel jealous or struggle with jealousy.

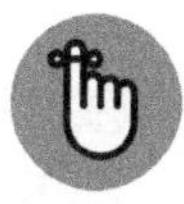
REMEMBER

Don't shame your partner for their jealousy.

And don't be hard on yourself for having jealous feelings. You live in a universe that indoctrinates you with scarcity fear and impossible, sometimes conflicting, standards around relationships. Don't add fuel to that dumpster fire.

Consider what it would be like to create an environment where you expect jealousy to arise in your kink relationships, and you welcome it as information about how well you are communicating and taking care of each other. The following sections explore this idea.

Good kinksters experience jealousy

Some people really do have a stronger inclination toward openness and experimentation. Even when their partners are excited about new possibilities or confess crushes, they experience very little jealousy. But the vast majority of us struggle with this concept.

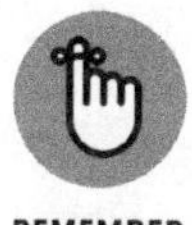
REMEMBER

Two of the keys to freedom from jealousy are simple:

>> Drop the self-judgment and perfectionism.

>> Drop the judgments of your partner.

WARNING

Telling a partner that they aren't brave enough or are too conventional for kinky play or exploration is the worst way to deal with a partner's scarcity fear or jealousy. If someone is doing this to you, they're out of line. If you're doing this to someone, you're out of line.

TIP

Use the resources in this chapter and in Appendix B to stop destructive behaviors around jealousy and figure out how to get the support you need.

Supporting your jealous partners

The best route toward dealing with jealousy is to *go toward the very difficult thing* rather than to deny, deflect, or retreat from it. If your partner is in deep distress, it's likely to activate your scarcity fear: *She is trying to take this away from me! She never supports me!* If you're the one in jealousy distress, you may be picking fights over something else or accusing your partner of things they haven't done in order to cover up your problematic jealous feelings.

TIP

Instead of jumping into denial, deflection, or blame, move toward your jealous self or toward your jealous partner with compassion.

MOVING CLOSER EXERCISE. This exercise gives you options for rejecting polarized behavior around jealousy. Instead of being judgmental or defensive, you and your partner can choose to be curious together. Here are a few statements and questions that show openness and interest in what's currently happening with your partner:

>> Oh honey, tell me more about this. I thought you were excited about going to this kink party.

>> I'm so glad you told me you're feeling this way. Thank you for trusting me.

>> I'm so sorry you've been carrying these feelings by yourself; it must have been really hard.

>> Do you know what set these feelings off? Was there some particular action that I took, or didn't take?

>> When did things start feeling off for you? Can you remember what was going on?

>> What do you need right now? How can I support you?

>> Let's just take a breath together. I know we can figure this out.

>> You're really doing a great job identifying what's going on for you lately. Your hard work is paying off.

>> I'm impressed that you've been able to share this. How can we work on it together?

The core practices that underly all of these statements are:

>> **DON'T JEER: J**udge, **E**scalate, **E**gg-on, or **R**idicule your partner for their emotional state.

>> **DO READ: R**eassure, **E**mbrace, **A**ffirm, and **D**e-escalate the situation by reading your partner's emotional state and responding with care.

ADDRESSING JEALOUSY TOGETHER. Taking on jealousy as a team project is a great way to avoid stigmatizing your partner or deflecting and denying that jealousy is even an issue. Working this exercise together will improve the likelihood of success.

Follow these steps together:

1. **Identify the things that trigger each of you.**

   Pinpoint what happens in your bodies so you can start to name these triggers and help each other address when jealousy is operating.

   Start to build a practice of breathing together when feelings of jealousy are being activated in you or your partner.

2. **Create a supportive shared catch phrase to use when you notice jealousy starting to take over the conversation.**

   Here are some examples:

   - Hey, I'm here for you. We're in this together.

   - It seems like you're being overtaken by the green monster — Roar!

   - Are you okay?

   Use humor. Break up the intensity by reminding each other that you've created a strategy together.

3. **Agree on supportive action to counter jealousy.**

   Determine what you can do for each other when one of you is experiencing a jealous episode. See if you can agree to do something that you love together. Is there a song, a dance, a snack, an ice-cream parlor, a walk, a hobby, a sport, or a goofy activity that can de-escalate the jealousy and bring you two together again?

   If one partner has identified specific triggers, create specific practices to counter those activating events — meaning what to do next.

4. **Possibly phone a friend.**

   Work together to identify excellent, resourceful friends to text or call when you're activated around jealousy. In the heat of activation, you can support each other by saying something like: "Maybe Angelique can support you right now. Do you want to reach out to them?"

Jealousy is often characterized as a natural way of protecting your relationship. But it's actually a learned behavior that fuels a system that says real relationships are once-in-a-lifetime, not kinky, and don't center pleasure. You don't have to buy into this. You can decide you don't like the way jealousy operates in your life and take a different path.

Coming Back from Broken Trust

Many of Jaime's coaching clients seek coaching after one or more partner has long suppressed their intimate and sexual needs in the relationship. Typically, this boils over in a way that breaches the agreements made within the relationship — one person has an emotional affair at work or has sex with a stranger. Perhaps someone is falling into a rabbit hole online, playing in a kink space that they can't figure out how to talk about in real life.

At the outset of the work, these clients are often in deep pain. They want to stay together, but the lies and buried desires operating between them are devastating. In this next section, we take you through possible routes for coming back from a breach of trust. While healing is always possible, staying together is not always the healing way forward.

Taking time to recover

An important consideration in deciding how to address a breach of trust is to give yourself time. Even though your relationship, and your life, may feel like it's in a state of desperate emergency, attending to this incredibly painful and disruptive event doesn't mean it needs to get solved in the next ten minutes.

TELLING YOUR STORY

When I've been lied to or betrayed by a lover or a partner, I need to tell the story. Over and over again. It's like my brain is trying to make sense of something it doesn't quite believe yet. I go through the events of finding out or receiving the disclosure. I put together timelines that led to the events. I re-create the story of the relationship with this new information inserted into the false narrative and dig around in all of the dishonesty that has brought me to this moment.

The only way to heal and to plot the right course for yourself to move forward is to really hear this story. And to hear it, you need to tell it because if you're like me — when I really love someone — I can deflect and deny and minimize what's happened to me. I can try so hard to see my lover's side of it that I can lose myself. Telling your story over and over again helps you hear it, shakes loose your denial, and clears a path to the next right step.

One of my favorite pieces of advice from a former AA sponsor is this: You can't will yourself to clarity. Clarity comes. **—Jaime**

And trying to get to resolution when speaking from a place of deep pain and betrayal almost never goes well or improves outcomes.

When you realize that you've been lied to or your partner has crossed a clear boundary, you may literally stop breathing. Being blindsided by a lie or series of lies can have cascading physical consequences. As always, everything is better with a breath or two. The emotional pain can create energetic devastation and even physical illness. Pay attention to what you're feeling. Allow yourself to take a time-out and recoup your energy.

De-escalating your sense of panic or distress can take time and support. Here are a few go-to support activities in times of a trust breach that may work for you:

>> Text, talk, and be with your closest friends.

>> Play your favorite soothing music or a survival anthem.

>> Eat good food. Determine whether a loved one can cook for you, or whether cooking for yourself will soothe you.

>> Spend some time doing your favorite physical activity. Maybe you enjoy a team or individual sport. Maybe you like dancing. Maybe heading to the gym or to the hills for a hike will take great care of you. Moving your body in joyful or connecting ways can be a great support.

>> Get your fan life on. Go to a concert. Go see your team fight to win. Go be with other fans.

>> Take in some art. Go see a favorite play, an exhibit, or a performance. Remind yourself of the bigger you beyond this really tough moment.

>> Consider bodywork. Bodywork, including massage, can help when a sense of betrayal is lodged deep. Look for a *trauma-informed practitioner* (a therapist, teacher, or bodyworker who has training in trauma.)

>> Hydrate and rest. Let us repeat: Hydrate and rest.

Telling your story over and over again is a clarifying practice.

Sifting through each person's needs

When a breach of trust has happened, you and your partner(s) may have wildly differing thoughts about what to do next. And that's okay. It's important to find a way to accommodate each other, while taking maximally good care of yourself. How can this be accomplished, especially if one person wants to talk through everything immediately while the other person needs time and space?

Not knowing what to do is a near universal problem, so don't be disheartened. You may think of the immediate aftermath of discovering a trust breach as triage in the emergency room. The nurses figure out right away what the most life-threatening situations are and address those first. Can't breathe? Let's get you a breathing tube. Bleeding profusely? Staunch that wound.

Speaking the truth about broken trust

Your broken trust triage statements may look something like this:

>> I can't talk to you right now.

>> I need to know exactly what happened right now.

>> I need (you) to find another place to stay.

>> I can't talk about this or work on this if you're seeing this person.

>> I need you to hold me and comfort me while I cry.

>> I really want to have make-up sex, but I think it's better if you don't touch me right now.

>> I need to cry and scream, and I can't do that with you here.

>> I can't hear an apology; you're just upset that you've been caught.

The person who has broken trust may have triage statements like these:

>> I need you to stay.

>> It's over with the other person; I need you to believe me.

>> I need to know you won't leave me.

>> I don't want to hurt you, and I want to keep seeing this person.

>> I love you the most, but I can't do what you want.

>> I have to go see them, but I'll be back.

You may notice that only I-statements are offered in the lists above. *I-statements* are simple declarations that lay out your truth and keep the focus on your feelings and experience.

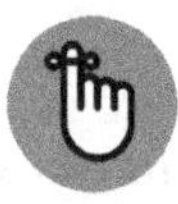

"I think you're a jerk" isn't an I-statement.

REMEMBER   I-statements are the way to go during a trust breach, but they can be very difficult to say. Being lied to or betrayed is the greatest generator of you-statements in the universe. "You need to stop seeing him. You screwed up big-time. You're the biggest liar that has ever lied."

If you can stay focused on I-statements in your triage moment, you'll feel better about yourself; and the decision-making process will be better. But if you do a bit of finger-pointing — you-statements — don't feel bad about yourself. Think about what you want here. Do you want to be self-righteous and just blow everything up? Then have at it. Sometimes a blowup is just part of the way through.

Determining what you need to do

To determine next steps after a trust breach, you may want to create an emergency plan to de-escalate the situation. Then, you can start to figure out what you need and whether mending this breach to move forward is even possible. Here's a simple guide for an emergency plan:

- >> Think about and create your specific needs and triage statements.

- >> Figure out how to get some space to breathe and to take in this new information. (See the earlier section, "Taking time to recover.")

- >> Make a short-term agreement.

Here's what the decisions may look like:

- >> I won't leave you, but you can't see them until we talk.

- >> We'll talk on Friday, after I've seen my therapist.

- >> We can get a mediator or therapist for our next conversation.

- >> I'm staying at my sister's this week while you stay here. Next week you'll need to find somewhere to stay while I come back.

- >> I'll try to think well of you while we're figuring this out.

- >> Any more lies or breaches in this period and I'm done.

Figuring out what's possible

Assessing whether recovery is possible, and whether a mended relationship of any kind, in any form is sustainable — may take some time. Things can't go back to the way they were prior to the breach. This experience will change you and the way forward, as it should. The question is, how? What's possible?

A mistake some couples make is rushing to apology and forgiveness rather than taking the time to poke around a bit in what has happened, how you feel, and what you need. Apologies and forgiveness declarations can be shortcuts when people are experiencing unbearable feelings and situations. People may also jump to an instant list of corrections or fixes because they don't want to stay in these feelings. Or they don't want to have to really talk about the problems that underlie the breach of trust. For example, you've been checking out of your relationship because you're work long hours, or your partner is having an emotional affair with a friend, or you're completely unavailable because you're the caregiver for your parents.

Sometimes structural changes in your relationship that pull your attention away from your partner or exhaust you aren't fixable. You have an infant to care for, or your partner has a parent who is dying, or you just got fired. If you're with someone over time, life unfolds, and life is demanding and messy. Inside all that messiness are unmet needs for both you and your partner. And if one of you has breached an agreement to get those needs met, it can be difficult to consider whether you can ever trust them again.

ACTIVITY

WHAT'S POSSIBLE? Taking a look at possible outcomes is an important way to navigate the road to recovery. Here are a few questions to ask yourself about whether recovery is possible:

» Is the person who has breached trust really taking responsibility for their actions?

   If yes, how are they doing this?

» What actions or changes are in place that demonstrate taking responsibility? Will these actually give you the space to heal and create a constructive way forward?

   If no, and if they are deflecting, blaming you or others, or minimizing what has happened, do you think they're capable of owning their part eventually?

» What indications do you have that your partner is capable of building a path toward owning their actions and making real amends?

» Do you have the capacity to forgive and re-establish trust? Do you think it's possible to learn from this, let go, and move forward with your partner?

   If yes, what are the conditions and actions that will make regaining trust possible?

   If no, do you want to build that capacity?

» What do you need in your life and your day-to-day connection to your partner to build on your capacity to trust?

You may not know the answers to these questions in the immediate aftermath of discovering a breach of trust. Take your time. Get support. These questions can be a guide as you move out of emergency mode and into considering your options or devising a plan to move forward.

A partner who has been unable to communicate honestly and be rigorous about assessing their own behaviors and shortcomings is unlikely to do better when opening your relationship to kink.

In this case, working hard to meet your partner's needs and affirming their right to pleasure may not be a positive step. Instead, unearthing new vulnerabilities and creating new intimate practices is likely to sow more chaos, deception, and pain.

Investigating the nature of the dishonesty

Sorting out what kind of lies are happening in your situation — its sources, functions, and impacts — may be helpful. Lies aren't justifiable, but many lies can be explained by looking at a lover's childhood burdens, trauma history, or patterns in past relationships. Having an explanation doesn't mean you need to excuse the lie or forgive the person breaching your trust. It's just helpful context as you consider what this means to you, your partner, and your relationship.

DISHONESTY DETECTIVE. This exercise provides a way to examine the lies you are dealing with more closely. Core questions to ask yourself or your partner include the following:

>> How is this lie connected to lies that my partner survived as a child?

>> How does this lie echo lies that I survived as a child?

>> How is this lie connected to survival mechanisms that my partner developed to take care of themselves when they were young and powerless?

>> What was the function of this lie? What did it hide?

>> Is this lie singular or part of a series of lies?

>> Is my partner ashamed of themselves on a fundamental level?

>> How does their shame mirror some of my shame — and does this amplify a sense of emergency right now?

>> Did our original agreements about our relationship hide or mask needs that my partner was ashamed to share?

>> How can this information help me figure out my next steps in recovering and taking care of myself?

As you recover from a trust breach, you may want to think about how or whether lies permeated your childhood and then continued as an adult. The devastation you feel at having someone abuse your trust may be very current, but it can also be amplified by abuses of trust in your past — in romantic or familial relationships.

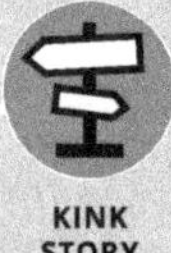

KINK STORY

NO ONE IS PERFECTLY TRUSTWORTHY

Thirteen years into our relationship, my boyfriend lied to me. We had some agreements about safer sex in our open relationship, and he broke our agreements and lied about it. We had come through a lot by then. He had gotten sober about five years before that, and I could see why he did it. He had a very controlling parent, especially around his sexuality. He grew up feeling very hemmed in emotionally and sexually. And he had to keep a lot of secrets just to be himself. This kind of sneaking around wasn't about me — it was just his trauma surfacing.

I knew what he did wasn't meant to hurt me and what he did really didn't endanger me or my health. In fact, if he had asked me, I would have easily agreed to changing our safer-sex guidelines. I think when he did it, he was in denial about it breaking my trust — like he wasn't even aware he was lying. But being lied to really hurt me, and undermined our relationship.

When people lie to me, I feel like they're trying to control my reality. And I resented being put in the position of his controlling parents in his internal story because that's the last thing I am or want to be. I let him know that lying was a deal-breaker for me and that he needed to figure out why he had lied and make a meaningful apology, or I was done.

And he did this. Which was wonderful, but what really struck me during the whole crisis was that I was not in crisis. I was so much less emotionally activated than I expected. And that was because in the whole of our life together — my boyfriend is wonderful. He's extremely trustworthy. He works so hard on his emotional growth, and he's generous and loving with me.

And this was a mistake. This mistake came out of work he still needs to do. It hurt me, but it wasn't about me, and I could see this clearly. Our forgiveness work of many years really held us in this period: I love imperfect him, and he loves imperfect me. And I can take care of myself and still believe in him when issues arise, because he takes responsibility for himself and he takes action to do better.

The deal is there are no guarantees. There is no perfect love out there. There is no "the one." There's just each of us struggling to act according to our values, and deeply caring for each other as best we can, as we grow. **—Dean**

Sorting out the past from the present is important work in order to stay present and assess. Refer back to Chapter 10 for more on this.

Recovery Is Possible

Against all odds and the intensity of your belief that everything is ruined and nothing will ever be the same, your relationship can recover. Nothing ever will be the same though. That part is true. In the aftermath of a breach of trust, you'll need to re-create many things: your ideas about yourself, your relationship with your partner (or partners), and your pathway forward. The following sections provide concrete tools for moving forward, into a place of rebuilding. Whether you have been the creator of, or the person impacted by a breach of trust, these tools can help you recover and move forward.

Making a great apology

Probably the single most important determinant on that way forward is whether the person who has broken trust is able to make a sincere apology.

Activist and writer Mia Mingus has created an excellent set of guidelines for making a great apology. If you can start here as partners, you have a lot in your favor in the recovery column. If you or your partner don't have the capacity to make an apology on these terms, get help. Seek friends or counseling resources that can help you get there. As a coach, Jaime has watched couples who have survived deep, disturbing betrayals come back from these abuses of trust — and a sincere, unreserved apology was the foundation of that recovery, every time.

Follow these key steps to apologize:

1. **Say you're sorry.**

    Simple. No equivocations. And "I'm sorry you feel hurt" isn't an apology. "I'm sorry I hurt you by telling you lies over many months." That's an authentic apology.

2. **Name the hurt.**

    Say what you did, plainly. "I told you lies over and over and made you think you were jealous or creating problems because I was trying to cover my tracks." No back-door discussion of your partner's issues, such as "I know this was hard on you because you're insecure."

3. **Name the impact.**

   Describe what effect your behavior had on the person you've hurt. "I know over time this made you question yourself, and it nearly drove you crazy." Or "I know that you can't trust me now and that I will have to work to regain your trust."

4. **Take responsibility by naming your actions.**

   Own what you've done; you alone are responsible for your actions. "I know I could have told you about my loneliness or my attraction to X, but I chose to hide those feelings and to start an affair instead."

   This following step is one of the most crucial parts of the apology to get right. Often, people who have broken a partner's trust will say something like, "things were messed up in the relationship for a long time," or "I didn't get here on my own." These statements may be true, but the responsibility for making a decision to break trust rests solely on the person taking that action. Making a true apology rests on your willingness to own your behavior — 100 percent — without reservations or footnotes.

REMEMBER

5. **Commit to stopping the behavior and not doing it again.**

   This is a big step. Many people find themselves apologetic when a breach of trust has happened, but changing behavior so that you're a more trustworthy partner is serious work. In a monogamous relationship, committing to stopping a behavior most often means that a partner ends an affair and usually all contact with the person.

   In kink worlds, committing to change can often be more complex. The breach may be about breaking an agreement like creating a more intimate relationship with a play partner than you initially agreed to. Accordingly, it may not mean ending the relationship with the person in question but adjusting practices or agreements. In a case like this, stopping the behavior means to stop telling lies and to recommit to adhering to your agreements, not necessarily removing the person from your intimate life.

When trust has been broken, figuring out the best way forward in a complex kink group of playmates and beloveds can be challenging. The important thing is to listen to the person or people whose trust has been betrayed to understand what their needs are going forward.

Rebuilding trust

Although a great apology is a crucial first step forward, it's just one step in a longer process. A core part of a long-term amends process is for the person who has betrayed trust to *sustain their commitment to honesty over time* and to consistently show up emotionally for the person or people they have harmed.

A sincere apology *plus* a commitment to honesty *plus* consistency *plus* time is the recipe for rebuilding trust. It's not rocket science; it's a very clear path. But that doesn't mean it's easily done.

Reconciliation and trust-building is a big job. When you have hurt someone, witnessing the impacts of your abuse of trust, over and over, is difficult. It's easier to check out of the situation — maybe staying late at work a lot or renovating a room in the house instead of sitting through painful dinners where your partner cries or is depressed.

Each person in the partnership or extended kink family should take great care of themselves during the recovery process. However, if you have breached an agreement, showing up for your partner (or partners) emotionally in the aftermath will be a crucial step on the path to mending your relationship.

Forgiving and letting go

Only you can decide if you can forgive and let go around a partner's abuse of your trust. Only you know what a healthy next step is for you. If you have a partner who is making a sincere apology and is undertaking a consistent amends process, you have an opportunity to rebuild trust. The question is — do you want to take it?

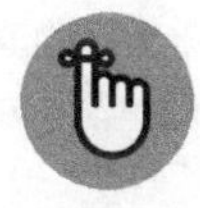

A truth about how difficult it is to forgive a partner who has lied to you is that it shakes the very foundation of your faith in yourself.

How could you not have known? How could you have put your trust in this person? How could this person who has seen you at your most vulnerable cast aside that sacred offering by deceiving you? Often the path to forgiveness of your lover starts with forgiving yourself. And that can be very difficult to do, especially if you're deflecting your anger at yourself by aiming it exclusively at your partner.

We don't want to be overly simplistic or fake-optimistic about this. Or campaign for forgiveness as though it's appropriate in every situation — *because forgiveness truly isn't appropriate in many situations.*

But forgiving a partner who has abused your trust can be an incredible gift *to yourself* under the right circumstances. Forgiving your partner after they have failed you — perhaps after they've showed you the worst side of themselves — demonstrates a kind of faith you may desperately hope others will extend to you.

Forgiveness is a gift for the worthy. And by that, we mean, those who are willing to go the hard way with you, and those who are willing to be just as fearless about their self-reflection as you are about yours.

You don't owe anyone your forgiveness. You get to decide who you share your intimate life with and what your bottom-line needs are. You can decide to forgive; you can decide to walk away. Nobody else has to like it or understand your decision. How you organize your intimate and sexual life is entirely, solely up to you.

Distinguishing Between Relationship Troubles and Abuse

Given the diversity of kink relationships — from lovers to play partners to hook-ups and many other kinds of kink intimates — figuring out when differences have become deal-breakers isn't easy. The following sections help you sort through your relationship values for clues to when you're at an ending point in any kind of kink relationship.

Being worn out and down: Deal breakers

Because kinksters often feel proud of their ability to discuss issues openly and co-create consent (see Chapter 3), recognizing when you are in a toxic or dangerous situation can be tough. People who are draining or abusive can hijack kink processes and language to their benefit, making you question your needs and your perceptions.

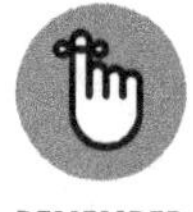

REMEMBER

Hallmarks of a truly terrible partnership — signs that it's time to say enough is enough — include the following:

>> You don't center your own needs in the relationship anymore; you don't even know what they are.

>> You're hooked on your partner's needs, moods, and reactions.

>> You keep having the same disagreement or fight without any progress or resolution.

>> You're spending more time in conflict than in kink exploration or growth.

>> You give in and abandon yourself repeatedly because you just want the conflict to be over.

>> Your partner is never wrong or rarely sees their part in any of these problems. You, too, may have become less likely to see your part.

>> Your partner never — or almost never — apologizes.

>> Your partner belittles you, privately or publicly.

>> Your partner refuses to get therapy, mediation, or any outside help individually.

>> It feels like you're just trying to survive.

>> Your relationship is impacting your mental and physical health.

>> All the work you're putting into this relationship is impacting your work-life and job security.

>> All the time you're pouring into this relationship is impacting your financial stability.

>> All the work you're putting into this relationship is making it difficult to stay connected to your friends; you're getting more and more isolated.

>> You feel like a failure.

>> Sometimes you're afraid of your partner or afraid for your well-being.

If you checked off more than two or three of the concerns on this list, it's time to think about your health and whether you've lost your way in this relationship.

Recognizing nonconsensual coercion

Coercion or manipulation in kinky scenes can be fun and sexy if that's what you are into. Jaime notes, as someone who enjoys this kind of play very much, that it's particularly arousing for her because she survived so much coercive manipulation as a young person trying to form her sexuality. So, like many kinksters, she plays in this territory with a trusted partner as a way to reclaim herself, and to turn the abuse on its head.

But what is *actual* nonconsensual coercion and manipulation? And how do you recognize it, especially among people who may have such a strong vocabulary around consent and are hiding in plain sight?

The basics of coercive control include:

>> **Undermining your self-confidence.** This may be subtle and take place over time. It may involve behaviors like questioning your clothing choices, making confusing or low-key negative comments about your friends or your work accomplishments, dissing or "joking" about something that matters to you like cooking, sports, or your art. It may extend to your kink play, with an encouragement on one hand, and then a harsh judgment or subtle negative comment on the other.

- >> **Isolating you.** A manipulator may slowly amp up their demands of your time and test your loyalty or commitment to the relationship by pitting your partnership against your key friendships. A master manipulator will cause conflict between you and your close friends perhaps causing breaches or friendship break-ups. They may try to move you away from your friends geographically to further isolate you. They may create problems with your job or even cause you to lose your job as a way to amplify your vulnerability.

- >> **Engaging in kink-specific coercive control.** An abusive Top may wear you down about your limits, suggesting that your growth as their bottom or a progression of your healing hinges on you dropping the limits that are meaningful to you. An abusive bottom may do the same, suggesting that when you are finally a *real Top* you'll do the things that *they* have defined for you.

A specific risk factor in kink worlds is that you are consensually working toward a vulnerable and exposed state with your partners. You have worked carefully to build trust and invest power in this person. The ecstatic states you've created together may be singular, like nothing you've ever experienced. A manipulator will count on this. The fear of losing this kind of connection may move you to accept things that feel slightly *off* or wrong in the beginning. Over time, you may be led to incrementally abandon yourself, until this person has power over your perception of events, and even your own needs.

Coercive control is very common

Depending upon the community you live in, it might be difficult to recognize coercive control because it is so common. In some religious communities, clerics are accorded a tremendous amount of power. And in some cases, men are invested with disproportionate decision-making power in relationships with women. In some university communities, top athletes or other superstars — including genius engineers, great actors or other artists — are lifted up as exceptional and even beyond reproach. In some workplaces, the CEO or founder or top performers may be beyond criticism.

Any community that extends so much power to one category of person or even one individual increases the potential for coercive control. Any community or institution that makes it harder for you to question decisions or speak up for yourself, erodes your ability to listen to your needs over time. Since your personal beliefs or wants don't matter in this system, why pay attention to them?

If you are in a kink community that idolizes certain leaders or kink players, take care of yourself. Sometimes people who are highly skilled or sought after for their particular kink practices have elevated social status. In some groups, people just worship the straight-up hotties. Observe people over time. Notice the well-being of their scene partners and lovers. Is everyone okay? Is it cool to ask questions about structures or practices that are in place in this social group? Is it acceptable to ask questions, period?

Being Isolated puts you in danger

If you are confused about whether you're experiencing coercive control, a key question to ask yourself is: has my world shrunk down to my partner's world? Here are a few specifics questions that may provide some clarity:

> » Does everything revolve around them — their ways of being, daily rhythms, and the things that are most important to them?
>
> » Do they have issues with my closest friends? Have they caused arguments or rifts with the people who love me best?
>
> » Is it difficult for me to have time with my friends alone? Or time with them at all?

If you answered yes to more than one of these questions, there's no confusion. You are with someone who is isolating you.

Get support. Some partners are somewhat controlling and can take responsibility for this when confronted. They are willing to own their behavior, get help, and change. And *many are not.* Figure out which lover, scene partner, or playmate you have. And take care of yourself.

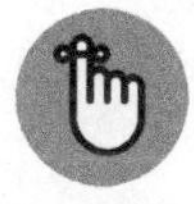

Creating physical and emotional distance from a manipulator is crucial because they are so good at clouding your judgment and confusing you. Their stock and trade is re-creating your social, emotional, and even physical environment so you feel lost or question your own beliefs. Getting out from under this requires cutting off their access to you. As Dua Lipa notes in her pop epic, *New Rules:* "If you're under him, you ain't getting over him."

Breaking up means creating distance — physical, emotional, social, and sexual — so that you can reset your emotional and intimate life and move into a more detached place of relating to this person.

Getting help

A few kink specifics are important to note if you find yourself needing help from someone who is manipulating and exerting coercive control.

» Predators count on stigma against kink to isolate you from help. If your partner is threatening to out you to a family member, friend or colleague, this is abuse.

» Your friends are your most important resource in times of crisis.

» Sometimes your *closest* friends are too close or invested in your relationship. Seek help from friends who can really listen and hear what you are going through. Stay connected.

» Breaking free from coercive control can take time. Because coercive control weakens your self-esteem and your support network over time, it can be difficult to break free. Remember that even if you've fallen out of touch, your friends will likely be relieved and glad to support you. Break your isolation. Keep reaching out.

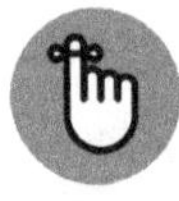

REMEMBER

Don't be hard on yourself for being in a controlling relationship. Keep seeking support even if your play partner or lover doesn't like it.

WARNING

If you are offering to help a friend in this kind of a situation, you are also at risk. Manipulators don't like threats to their control. They can also use kink stigma to get you to back off. They can call your workplace, discredit you as a kink player in the scene, or even try to use state authorities against you.

Your friend may also be resistant to your help as a result of being thoroughly manipulated by their abuser. It may be difficult to watch what is happening and still stay connected to your friend. So we recommend the following for those who are trying to help someone under coercive control:

» Take very good care of yourself.

- Talk to others about what you are going through.

- Keep an eye on your own sense of depression or anxiety.

- Take breaks if you need to.

- Protect your foundational relationships.

- Rally your friends if the abuser tries to target you in some way.

» Let your friend know you are not going anywhere. Even if they cut you off. Even if they are angry with you. Let them know you respect their decisions *and* you remain deeply concerned about their well-being. Let them know you are still there if they ever want to talk.

WARNING

Abuse isn't a natural part of kink life; it is pervasive to social and intimate life in the U.S.. Despite our best efforts, kinksters can't entirely escape its reach.

TIP

If you are suffering from coercive control or any other kind of violence in your kinky world, your best action is to tell yourself the truth and, at the very least, confide in one person who cares about you. *Telling one supportive friend can make all the difference.* And that is a true kink value.

4

Living Your Best, Sustainable Kinky Life

Chapter **13**

Finding Kink Community and Great Play Spaces

Kink community spaces come alive through the people who organize them — the kinksters who show up in the space, and the specific community agreements and kink culture that forms around that alchemic mix. When you find the organizers, community members, and ground rules that align with your values, you will find your people and play partners.

This chapter offers ideas for finding your kinky people — building community online and in person, and identifying the play spaces that are right for you. We also show you how to start doing the sometimes difficult work of overcoming the stigma or social anxiety, which could be holding you back from getting what you want.

Getting Online

Often, the first way kinksters put themselves out there is on the Internet. For some people, it's the only way that ever works. Connecting online has much to offer. You can tightly control your anonymity, and you can dip your toes in the sexy waters without having to wade in too deep. You can also explore at entirely your own pace.

Dating apps and social networks

For much of the world, dating apps are primarily for finding dates. Once users are partnered up, they tend to drop off these platforms. But for kinky people, dating apps and other social networks provide a space to connect, try on new identities or desires, flirt, and find playmates, regardless of relationship status.

Here are three prominent kink-friendly dating spaces online:

- » **FetLife** (https://fetlife.com). Since 2008, FetLife has been a major digital gathering place for U.S. kinksters of all genders, sexualities, and fetishes. It features forums for kink discussion, events pages for your area, and the ability to browse and flirt with other users.

- » **Feeld** (https://feeld.co). Feeld started its life in 2014 as a dating app for organizing threesomes, particularly for couples seeking a third. But it quickly evolved into an app for all kinds of people who may have felt hemmed in by the culture of mainstream dating apps. This website is great for polyamorous people, people exploring their genders and sexualities, and kinksters.

- » **Recon** (www.recon.com). For gay and bi men (and everyone who plays with gay and bi men), Recon is a specifically kink-focused social networking app, allowing users to see those around them with the same interests.

Many kinksters find success networking on non-kink dating apps just by putting their kink desires on their profiles. For some people, using mainstream dating apps like Tinder (https://tinder.com), Hinge (https://hinge.co), OKCupid (www.okcupid.com), or Bumble (https://bumble.com) works well. This is similar for the apps centered on queer women, like Lex (www.lex.lgbt) and HER (https://weareher.com).

In some spaces, users can write that they're looking for kinky partners right up front in their profile. For example, Lex is structured primarily around personal ads, where you can describe exactly what you're looking for. But remember that when these apps are location-based like Tinder, you never know who may see your profile — your boss or your cousins maybe — so some users save the specifics of their desire for user-to-user conversations to preserve their privacy.

Many of the gay and bi male-centered apps like Grindr (`www.grindr.com`), Scruff (`www.scruff.com`), and Jack'd (`www.jackd.com`) allow you to search by hashtags that can be used for specific kinks. You can even search this way without putting your kinky keywords out in the open as part of your profile.

Whether kink-specific or not, all of these social platforms include large numbers of users who are primarily looking to connect in real life. But they're also for people who just want to talk online. Some of these folks want to chat and share the intimate contents of their fantasies, while others want to talk dirty, try on new kink personas, and role-play.

TIP

If you're only looking for online connection so that you can explore your kinks in relative safety or anonymity, say that up front. Write it in your profile or tell people early in a conversation. It'll mean that not everyone whose profile you're drawn to will be a match. But the more clearly you articulate what you're looking for, the more likely you are to find people who can support your exploration.

Sharing erotica

Another way that kinksters connect online is through sharing grassroots erotica. Many people explore their kinks by reading, writing, and sharing stories. These range in length from a few paragraphs to say, an ongoing series that is published over the course of decades. Communities form around this art through praising comments, circulating favorite stories, and writing prompts for friends.

The great thing about these communities is that there is a high value in really taking care of each other. Sometimes this means helping another kinkster find what they like with story tags or avoid what they don't like with content warnings. Occasionally, these relationships cross over into taking care of real-life needs too, like fundraising for a beloved author to get needed medical care or a new laptop for writing.

Here are three online spots to check out for grassroots kinky stories:

>> **Literotica** (`www.literotica.com`). For anyone who has ever searched the Web for erotic stories, Literotica is always toward the top of search results.

Since 1998, its community of over two million users have amassed more than half a million stories, poems, essays, illustrations, and audio recordings, so there's truly something for everyone.

>> **Archive of Our Own** (AO3; `https://archiveofourown.org`). One common type of online erotica is fan fiction, which takes characters or real people from existing media properties like novels, movies, TV shows, and bands and casts them in original stories. Not all of these stories are kinky or erotic, but many of them are. The pre-existing relationship the writers and readers have with the characters act as an amplifier for their arousal. Fan fiction has sometimes come under attack because of the questions it poses about copyright law. So in 2008, a group of mostly women and queer activists launched a non-profit, The Organization for Transformative Works (OTW), to host a fan fiction archive and do the legal advocacy necessary to keep AO3 open and accessible. Today, the website hosts over fifteen million stories based in over seventy thousand fandoms.

>> **Nifty Erotic Story Archive** (www.`nifty.org`). For stories that are specifically lesbian, gay, bisexual, and transgender, Nifty has long been a central hub with subdivisions for specific kinks and fantasies like Dom/sub, first time, and urination. Nifty welcomes stories that are original as well as fan fiction.

WARNING

Many erotica authors go to great lengths to separate their online persona from their real name. Being identified with kinks or fantasies that people may not understand can cause real risk in real life (see Chapter 14).

KINK AND FRIENDSHIP ON BABYLON 5

I was exploring kink through fan fiction and erotica long before I ever had access to actual in-person play — maybe even before I knew what the word "kink" meant. This has been really important to figuring out my kinks, but it has also given me lifelong friendships.

There is one person I originally met through our shared excitement over amateur kinky romance novellas based on the sci-fi drama, *Babylon 5*. I've never met her in person, but she has been a kind of pen pal and confidant for over twenty-five years. We've known each other through marriages, divorces, the births of children, trying triad polyamory formations, and so many job changes. When I need to talk about something that I'd prefer not to delve into with anyone I interact with in person on a regular basis, I know I can always write to her and she'll give me a listening ear and an honest response. **—Jack**

Getting Offline

You can absolutely build a fulfilling kink life entirely online or in the private confines of one-on-one relationships with people you meet on the Internet. But if and when you find yourself ready to for more in-person spaces, you can start looking for opportunities to connect to community offline. In this section, you can find all the different in-person spaces kinksters gravitate toward to talk about their kinks and meet friends and play partners.

Finding non-sexualized spaces

If you're looking to discover more about your kink, but you'd like to do so in a non-sexualized or less-sexualized social space, there are many options for you.

>> **Munches.** A munch is a purely social gathering of kinky people. They can take place in dungeon spaces or other spaces owned by kink groups, but they can also happen in public, at restaurants, bars, or coffee shops. The idea is to build community and allow people to meet and talk without the pressure of playing immediately. For many people getting out there in the kinky world for the first time, a munch is a great, casual first stop. Fetlife keeps a calendar of announcements for munches.

>> **Classes.** Many kink organizations prioritize community education so that everyone can discuss how to get what they want safely. To that end, they often offer classes and demonstrations (or demos), which can also provide an opportunity to socialize and network. The classes are often popular for folks who are interested in highly complex kinks like rope play, or sadistic practices that require close attention or special skills (see Chapter 4 for more information on rope play and sadism).

>> **Kink-adjacent gatherings.** Kink-specific events aren't the only places to find kinky people. One example is the increasingly popular cuddle parties that are hosted all over the country, where people come together for non-sexual comfort and connection. If you are starting to explore kink desire, gatherings like these can be a place to find kinksters and other likeminded people.

>> **Socials.** Although you may often feel isolated, kinksters are everywhere — in every town, city, and region of the world. So, wherever you are, you may have luck making connections in non-cruising social spaces. Organizations like Open Social (`https://opensocial.club`) focus on encouraging friendship and can help you to build your social world.

>> **Conferences.** Finally, political and activist spaces focused on sexual liberation can be a space to build community and change the world. One example is the Leather Leadership Conference (`www.leatherleadership.net`) in Los Angeles, which seeks to empower kink leaders and educators. Another is Creating Change, the annual conference of the National LGBTQ Task Force, which annually includes a track of programming on sexual freedom and liberation.

The biggest clearinghouse of in-person events for kinksters in the United States is on Fetlife (`https://fetlife.com`). Check out the website's calendar interface and search according to your interests and geography. If you're chatting with other kinksters in your area virtually, on dating apps or other online spaces, you can also ask them about their favorite local events.

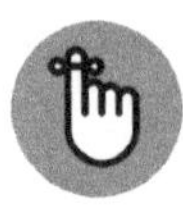

Always ask yourself how far you'd be willing (and able) to travel to connect with people in the space you're looking for. It's not unusual to find people at kink events who have driven great distances or taken trains, planes, and ferries to find the community they're seeking.

Play parties and dungeons

Perhaps the most iconic kink space is the dungeon. Many people create private playrooms in their own homes to function as their dungeon. There are also established clubs and play spaces, public or semipublic spaces that house a cache of tools, toys, and furniture that can be employed for kink scenes. Many dungeons have big open play areas where the more exhibitionist-inclined kinksters may play out their scenes, as well as smaller zones that pairs or small groups of people may use if they'd like just a little bit of privacy.

The dungeon in our city of Washington, DC is called *The Crucible*. It's open every weekend, sometimes for open play and other times for specific events, including education and demos. They often offer play nights hosted by one of the many local kink groups that focus on a specific style of play or a specific demographic audience. Formal and informal spaces like this are all over the country, from big cities to rural areas.

Read the room!

In all of these kink play spaces, ground rules or operating agreements will be posted by the host or Dungeon Master. Read them. Internalize them. If you don't understand them, ask people in charge for clarification. They will be happy to help. Or ask a cute kinkster you've observed in the space. What a great way to introduce yourself!

LEATHER EVENTS, CONTESTS, CLUBS, AND SPACES

In Chapter 4, the basics of the Leather community are discussed. It's an enduring kinky subculture that uses specific visual props and references, including a lot of leather, and builds complex sexual and social worlds and family structures.

Leather worlds are so vibrant and expansive — like the Leather clubs that grew of motorcycle club culture and act as a kind of fraternal/sororal space. There are also annual contests that are patterned after beauty pageants, in which Leather people show off their gear and skills and win titles. You can find endless parties, fundraisers, educational events, annual conventions, and Leather-specific munches.

For example, the Leather community may offer an early stop on their journey before finding a particular group of kinksters — say, people who are obsessed with rubber, or foot fetishists for example. Others will continue to spend time in Leather spaces because Leather community is open and inviting and may allow you to connect with likeminded people, even if you never become Leather-identified yourself.

Whether you're in a space where kink scenes are actively unfolding or not, entering unfamiliar territory will go much more smoothly if you try your best to match the energy of those around you. Some kink spaces may be loud and chatty. People may be making jokes and laughing, and if they are, then by all means, feel free to join in. But if the mood is quiet and reverent, don't be the only person speaking above a whisper and disrupting the vibe.

Dungeons aren't the only play spaces that may be available in your area. Here are some other possibilities.

- **Bars.** Some bars host kink nights where attendees are encouraged to wear fetish outfits, and there may even be limited forms of play. For example, a bar may hold a spanking night where spanking implements are provided, and people can use them on each other.

- **House parties.** Though it may take more work to find and get invited to private house parties, these occur all over the country, especially in places that may not be large enough to sustain a local dungeon.

- **Conventions.** Some of the biggest kink spaces are annual conventions that take place mostly in hotels or resorts. These events may include educational opportunities and demos, a marketplace where you can buy specialty kink tools and clothing, dance parties, leather contests (see Appendix B), and an opportunity to network with kinksters from all over who may host play in their hotel rooms.

>> **Bathhouses.** For gay and bi men, bathhouses have long been a mainstay for making sexual and community connections. Bathhouses generally have both wet and dry areas, with the wet areas including hot tubs, steam rooms, or saunas; the dry areas provide space for play. Some bathhouses are equipped for elaborate kink play and even some that aren't have devoted kinky followers who engage in all kinds of play there.

Not all kink community revolves around dungeons or play spaces. Groups of kinksters are everywhere and engaged in all kinds of actives, from book clubs to quilting, and even athletics (see nearby sidebar).

Adhering to laws and rules

Many kink spaces have faced intense scrutiny from law enforcement and disapproving neighbors, which means they have had to work extra hard to stay within the letter of the law. Many dungeons, for example, are set up as membership institutions, requiring a formal registration process in order to get in the door. For places where penetrative sex is taking place as part of play, they often can't allow alcohol or any sort of drugs to be consumed on the premises.

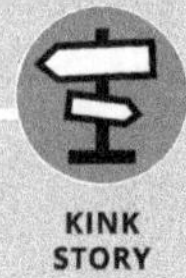

KINK STORY

THE P-SQUAD AND DOMMING IN PUBLIC

In my 30s, I was playing full-contact football as a member of the DC Divas, a professional women's football team. For me, the brotherhood that I found with my teammates really allowed me to grow, play, and stretch certain parts of myself. Football offered a unique opportunity for those of us butch/masculine of center — a place to be accepted and validated openly, on the field and off.

There was a crew of us that definitely earned the name, The P-(for P*ssy) Squad. Once it was said, (half) jokingly . . . it stuck! The feeling of freedom, to be able to carry all of myself, wherever I went, was immeasurable. We definitely didn't shy away from showing up (anywhere) as warriors, gentlemen, and thieves on a particular mission, all at once!

Though my kink life is mostly private, the experiences I've had at events or parties have also been important to me. Domming in public, I get to take up space as a Black, butch, queer, masc, nonbinary person. It pushes on freedoms I have every right to explore and claim as my own. **—M'Bwende**

There may also be rules about forms of kink play that can't be allowed due to local laws. This often includes things like blood or scat play that could be construed as a health hazard.

As you step into these kink spaces, note that they are important community institutions. It's up to you, and everyone, to uphold their guidelines so they can carry on without being shut down due to legal violations.

Paying attention to access

While kinksters may work to ensure that anyone and everyone is welcome at their events, not all kink spaces are equally accessible to all people. For example, some kink spaces are created explicitly for people who come with a partner and do not allow singles.

Some spaces are run as small businesses and may require a membership fee. However, even a small fee may mean some people can't afford it. Some kink retreats take place by the beach on Caribbean islands that require plane tickets and expensive hotel reservations. If that's in your budget, there are many kinksters who report fantastic experiences at these retreats. But the downside is that only those of a certain socioeconomic class get to be a part of it.

Beyond money, there can be issues around identity documents. To become a member of some dungeons or get on the list for some individual events, everyone must present a valid government-issued identification (ID). Community members may be vulnerable in different ways that make obtaining ID difficult, including some people immigrating or transitioning gender.

Denying access to certain groups can also happen on a slightly more subtle level. Many BIPOC kinksters report feeling alienated from kink groups that host parties where there are few people of color, of if they are the only BIPOC person in attendance. Others have been driven away when groups host parties with culturally appropriative themes, like "geisha nights" or "harem parties" that are not being organized by kinksters of that heritage. In these cases, BIPOC people may not be intentionally excluded, but a message is still being sent that some cultures are to be exoticized and used as set dressing.

Yet it is a common experience of kinky life that many kinksters have to build groups and spaces that meet their specific needs. While the kink community champions openness and accessibility, not everyone or every space has the capacity to create welcoming or culturally congruent experiences for all of the differing identities and needs in the community.

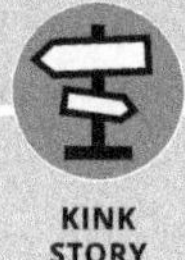

I HAD TO THROW MY OWN PLAY PARTIES

I've worked with a lot of Asian American advocacy groups, and my first race-specific organizing project was having this big fight about race with a gay boy circuit party. The organizers wanted to throw a "Year of the Dragon" party with a racist pan-Asian theme. When they refused to listen to the voices of people of color, I launched a campaign calling them out and educating the LGBTQ+ community about racism.

This was in the early 2000s and people had even less consciousness around racism than they do now. Looking back, it was a key political moment but then, I was just mad about the racist theme. I didn't realize my effort was going to help me meet other queer Asian activists all over the country. I also didn't understand that this conflict would lead me to throw my own play parties that were just for people of color and sometimes just for Asian Americans. **—Asha**

Over the past 30 years, many new kink spaces have emerged that make room for and affirm more genders, races, cultures, sexual orientations, kinky passions, and particular fetishes. You might start your journey of discovery thinking that you will never find others with your particular obsession or social or cultural need within the kink community. Eventually, you may be surprised to find a space that is exactly what you are longing for, or you may decide to create your own.

Becoming the host of your own kink space or party is an enormous responsibility (see the nearby sidebar, "I Had to Throw My Own Play Parties"). Suddenly you are in charge of creating and sustaining a consent agreement shared among everyone in attendance.

Going to someone's home

The last in-person space to discuss is private homes. Whether it's yours or the home of someone you've met on the Internet, sharing private space with people you don't know well comes with risk.

There are many communities that do this routinely, and the shared sense of responsibility among the group to ensure one another's safety is extremely powerful. But things do happen. People may experience theft, physical harm, and emotional abuse.

One consideration for your safety is whether you're meeting one-on-one or in a group. For many, even a small group may feel more comfortable than being alone one-on-one, especially for a first-time meeting. A private dungeon party in someone's home means there are more people to witness your play and ideally hold the host accountable.

Here are a few questions to ask yourself when considering going to someone's home for play.

>> Do I feel more comfortable going to someone's space if I can bring a friend, or if the scene involves more than two people?

>> Do I feel more comfortable meeting a group of people if I've seen photos, know their names, or have contact information for all involved?

>> Do I feel comfortable with the host of a private group event sharing my photo, name, and/or contact information with all involved?

>> Do I feel more comfortable having someone in my space or going to someone else's space?

>> If someone is coming to my space, where am I keeping my wallet and other valuables?

>> If I'm going to someone else's space, do I need to bring my wallet and ID?

>> Is there someone I can tell about my plans just in case something bad happens to me?

>> Is there someone I can share my location with on my phone so they can see where I am?

>> Are there activities I want to do with this person but that might be better saved for after a first play date? Activities like being bound or sensory deprivation come with a higher level of risk.

Fighting the Nerves

Putting yourself out there and asking people to play inherently involves rejection. If you make attempts to connect, you will be rejected, at least some of the time. And that can be hard on your self-esteem. It may tank your willingness to try again. The fear of rejection might make you hesitant to put yourself out there at all, but the reward can be so worth the risk. This section has some tips and tricks to help you through.

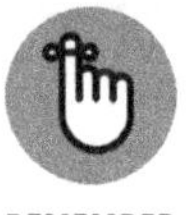

Everyone gets rejected, even the hottest people you can imagine. Experiencing rejection puts you in very good kinky company.

Getting ready

For some people, not knowing what to wear can be enough to keep you from going to the function at all. But don't let that get in your way! Check the event dress code, if there is one.

Also, be sure to check the space's rules on footwear, which may be listed separately from the dress code for an individual event. Some places may have rules against sneakers and others may not allow stilettoes. But the rules should be clearly posted on the website or event posting.

If you really don't know what to wear, all black is always a good option.

Figuring out how to approach

There was a time in some kink communities when you had to really know the protocol before you could approach someone to play. For example, if you were interested in a sub (submissive) who was in a Leather family (see Appendix A) and there was someone else present who was higher than that person in the family's hierarchy, you needed to go to that person for permission to even ask about connecting. Many of these traditions have loosened over time, particularly with the advent of the Internet, but that has left many newcomers, especially those who are early in their exploration journey, without a clear sense of how to enter and behave in these spaces.

The truth is that how you approach going into a new kink situation is largely the same as how you approach any new situation. Be polite. Be respectful. You may want to smile or otherwise signal your interest and good intention. It also pays to have done a little exploration into your own flirtation style.

FLIRTATION STYLES. Here are a set of questions to ponder when considering your flirtation style.

>> Do you feel comfortable being clear and asking for what you want directly?

>> Do you feel turned on by asking for what you want directly?

>> Do you imagine you would be excited and respond well to being flirted with by someone else, clearly and directly?

>> Do you feel more comfortable asking someone to play who you've met a few times or at least had a conversation with? Or are you open to anyone, regardless of whether you've ever seen them before?

>> Do you like an evening's-long build-up of flirtation before play happens — maybe starting with making eyes at each other across the room? Or do you want a longer period of getting-to-know-you that might include several meet-ups? Is that part of your kink?

For many kinksters, a long-drawn-out flirtation like a cat and mouse game may be their kink. It may be all they actually need for fulfillment. For others, a period of exchange of information and interest is just something they have to navigate to get where they really want to be.

Bring a friend. So much about kink life, and life in general, is easier when you're not going it alone. Having a kink confidant or wing person to go to new spaces with can make you feel more relaxed, safer, and help you to have more fun.

Trying out volunteering

If you feel uncomfortable attending a play party as a relative newbie (or as an observer who isn't sure whether they actually want to play or not), having a volunteer role can help to calm you down and build confidence in your place in the event. It also shows the people around you that you're serious about building the community and willing to put in the effort.

If there are classes, parties, or other kinds of spaces that you have access to, they often need volunteers. Giving your time and being of service to the community can give some kinksters a feeling of arousal and satisfaction in and of itself. And kink spaces always need service providers to keep activities on track.

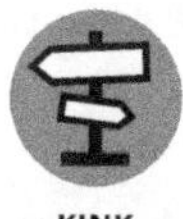

I think I had some naiveté when I finally started experimenting. My first-ever kink experience — I liked it so much that it freaked me out! I had been watching BDSM porn since I was really young, but I didn't realize how different that was from navigating kink in real life. My first-ever kink dynamic was with someone who was a semi-professional Dom. I didn't realize that kink could be like a drug. I didn't realize how the intensity of the experience could be addictive. That kind of got really mixed up because I didn't have a strong sense of my boundaries at that point; I didn't have structure. So, I got very, very swept up and fell into a level of intensity and some unsustainable dynamics for my well-being. **—Gina**

Finding partners who are excited to go with you at the same pace as you will be crucial to your kink enjoyment.

Knowing when to leave the party

When exploring kink spaces, the most important thing you can do is listen to your own instincts. If you feel unsafe or you're so nervous that you're not having a good time, that's your inner self giving you a warning sign that's worth paying attention to. There will always be more opportunities to play — more parties, more invitations to people's homes, and more spaces to explore. So if you have to cut some short, don't worry that you'll never have another chance.

On the other hand, there can be a level of nervousness that calls you to move through it. Your kink desires may feel a little bit scary; and for many, that's even part of the fun. Deciding when your nerves should be embraced and when they're telling you to leave may not always be easy, but you can develop the ability to see where that line is drawn.

When you listen to yourself and follow the path that feels right to you, so much joy and connection is possible.

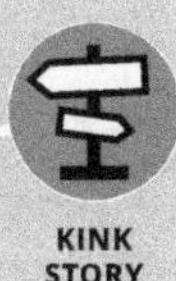

I CAN MAKE MY OWN STARS ALIGN

Just before I graduated college, I interned in San Francisco. The first thing I did was go to an Exiles meetings, which is a queer women–centered kink group in the Bay area. They had social get-togethers and skills-building workshops. I went to a couple of meetings, but I was excited for a real play party.

Of course, I was "fresh meat" — I had this hilarious moment where I found myself basically in a circle of five experienced women asking me what I'm into, and me having no idea whatsoever!

That night, two people co-Topped me. I negotiated the scene to include impact play and spanking, and I don't even know what else I said, but I was very brave; and it was very terrifying to be surrounded by all these high-skilled Tops!

I remember being in a very expensive cab ride back to Berkeley that night, and I felt great. I had only just come out as queer in college and been sexually active for a few years and now was adding this BDSM piece! I rode home feeling so lucky and so proud of myself that I'd made the stars align to get exactly what I wanted. **—Asha**

Chapter **14**

Coming Out Kinky

Claiming your love of kink and living openly is undeniably powerful. But you don't have to come out to live an empowered and satisfying kinky life. Let's say that again for the people in the back: You can live a great kinky life in private, or even in the confines of your own mind and solo practices.

You're the only person who knows what's going to work for you in a culture that is often highly judgmental of kink, stigmatizing and rejecting kinksters. Only you can weigh all the the pros and cons of coming out to make decisions that take the best care of you and your beloveds.

Being "out" as a kinkster is layered. You can be "out" in some spaces and "closeted" in others. It's an exercise in balancing risk and taking great care of yourself. Take your time as you discover the balance that is going to work for you.

Secrets make you sick. Privacy can make room for you to be more of who you are.

So an important question is what's the difference between secrets and privacy? Here are a couple of definitions to consider:

» A *secret* is often forced upon you by someone with power over you. Secrets leave you queasy, worried, fretting, or afraid.

> *Privacy* is something you set up and secure for yourself: "I can decide when and where to tell my story. I can take care of myself and my loved ones." Privacy feels like you are the boss of your life.

This chapter helps you consider what coming out kinky means to you and how to build the support you need to live a great kinky life. Here, you'll find supportive tips and stories as you think about to what degree you're ready to come out — to yourself, to a potential date, to family members, to your book group or rugby team, to coworkers, or whomever.

Coming Out Is a Process

Coming out is a process, not an event. You come out first to yourself, and then take a lifelong journey of sharing your truth and your desires with others in many different situations.

Similar to coming out LGBTQ+ or polyamorous, coming out kinky throws people into intimate territories in your life. It may expose you to hostile or inappropriate questions. It might put you in the path of someone's prejudice or negative judgments.

However, unlike coming out LGBTQ+ or polyamorous — when you are broadly revealing to another person the kinds of romantic partners you seek or the way you want to form your social and familial life — coming out kinky informs people about your intimate and sexual practices.

Jaime notes, looking back on her coming out journey:

> When I came out as a lesbian, people thought I was a non-conformist or even an outcast; when I came out polyamorous, people were widely confused and some branded me a slut. But coming out kinky was an even greater risk to my social and professional life — some people concluded that I was sick or dangerous.

Ask yourself: how important is it for a casual friend, a party organizer, your landlord, or your coworker to know?

In some of these cases, coming out may mean you're claiming your true self and connecting in a social space that is meaningful to you, and it can build joy and self-esteem. In others, it might mean that you're exposing yourself to someone with the power to shape your life or your future prospects, and it can bring risk and economic repercussions.

AFTER MISPLACED TRUST, I'M MUCH MORE PRIVATE

A few years ago, I had a coworker who was watching a lot of kinky movies like *Secretary* and *Fifty Shades of Grey*. We were pretty close — I would have called her a friend more than a coworker — so I thought it was okay to confide in her that I dominate and flog my wife in our sex life.

The following Monday, our boss called me into his office first thing in the morning. When I entered the room, the HR director was also sitting there. My heart sank; I immediately knew I was being fired, but I had no idea why. They both acted like it was obvious, but when I asked for clarification, they said they had become aware that I was talking about committing spousal abuse with coworkers. For a second, I had hope that this was actually going to work out because, obviously, there had never been any abuse at all between me and my wife. It was all consensual kink and fantasy play. But then they told me that they did not want any more information about "the abuse" for fear that it could implicate them in my "crimes" and that being fired wasn't up for negotiation.

After I walked out, I called my kinky confidantes. My heart went into some kind of self-protective dissociation mode for the rest of the day. My friends were really there for me, and my wife was totally supportive and appalled. But over the next several days and weeks, I went through so much emotionally. It made me question whether my kinks were, in fact, abuse or at least some kind of sign that I was mentally ill. I'd never thought that before but losing a job because of it was also such an extreme consequence of casual conversation about kink, and it really shook me up.

In the end, I know the truth of my heart. I know that I love my wife and that the way we play is the opposite of abuse; it's an incredible expression of our love. But being fired because I came out about my kinks to someone I thought I could trust has been one of the most traumatizing things I've ever experienced. It's made me a much more private person. **—Anonymous**

The following sections may help you sift through the risks and rewards of coming out kinky.

Coming Out to Yourself

The most important person to come out to about being kinky is you. If being kinky is important to who you are and how you want to pursue intimacy and love, then the most important person to tell is yourself.

Here are some questions to ask yourself about who you are:

>> Have you often fantasized about kinky play or scenarios?

>> Do you enjoy watching porn or reading erotica that includes kink?

>> Do you feel like your intimate life is lacking because nothing approaches the kind of intensity and arousal you feel about your potential kinks?

>> Has failing to pursue kink in your intimate life felt strange, confining, or like you were living a lie?

>> Have you felt like you had to hide all these feelings to fit into your friendship or social circle?

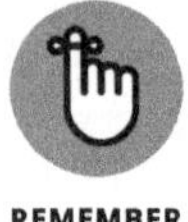

REMEMBER

Being true to yourself isn't overrated. Living your life openly among family, friends, and colleagues is enlivening. You spend less time worrying, sifting, and creating a narrative for others. You spend more time stretching into all the amazing possible ways to be you.

When you come out to yourself, you're opening a door inside you that can now lead outward: to new ways of being, new love, and a new dynamic, vibrant life. Refer back to Chapter 5 if you need help with discovering or defining your kinks.

Considering a Scene Name

There are many kinksters who are very prominent in Leather or otherwise kink communities who are only known by their *scene names*. This is a moniker a player has crafted for themselves in order to be proudly out and even in leadership in a kink community, while creating a firewall between that persona or set of practices, and their familial and professional life.

In some cases, a kinkster's legal name is widely known by many, and in others, there's an impenetrable divide between one's daily and professional life, and one's kink connections and activities.

Sometimes, a kinkster is protecting the identity and privacy of non-kinky family members. Sometimes, they are protecting a life in say, the clergy or big business where investors might have a negative reaction to discovering the scenester's kink life.

All of that is to say, creating a scene name and separating your kink from your "civilian" life might be something to consider. If you have family and assets to protect, this may be a practical route to take.

Being Out Isn't the Same Risk for Everyone

Once you come out kinky, you can't take it back. Whoever you've come out to is holding information that could be harmful to you in certain contexts. This may depend on where you live, what kind of legal and policing systems are in place, and what kind of social power and vulnerabilities your family holds. Coming out kinky can be like putting a weapon in your friend or coworker's hand that they don't understand or know how to control.

Coming out kinky isn't the same risk for every kinkster in every locality. It's not the same risk for people depending on your social and economic status, gender, race, citizenship, religious community, and so on. Kinksters have lost their jobs. Parents have had their custody challenged by hostile family members or have had neighbors call child protective services on them.

You know what risks you are carrying in terms of average, daily discrimination and violence. Being visible about your kink life adds a layer of vulnerability. Be sure you fully understand your family's vulnerabilities before thinking about coming out socially. Protect them by thinking through all of the possibilities.

Building Community: The Joy of Coming Out

Next to you, the most important people to come out to in your kink life are your close friends, partners, and your crushes. Coming out kinky is about connection, community, and often, release. Letting go of your reservations — having navigated your safety needs — can be wildly freeing and joyful.

Coming out can help you carve out the space for expansive kink possibilities. A common experience for kinksters as they come out is that they find people they are close to are also kinksters. In the past, all of this information had been hidden.

In this section, you can sift through questions about who, how, where, and when to come out. You can also assess whether you have enough support in your life to come out. And if not, you can find out how to build a kink-positive pod of confidantes and supportive activities.

Figuring out who tell

Building the kink life you want starts with finding the community you want. At the outset of your coming out considerations, focus first on the who:

1. Who do I want to tell?

2. Who am I excited to tell?

3. Who is a low-to-no-risk tell?

    - They are kinky themselves.

    - They hold no social or economic power in my life.

    - They hold strong principals around sex, justice, and freedom of expression.

4. Who matters to me?

5. How might coming out create an opportunity to be closer?

When we think about the people who have been the most supportive to us about kink, they didn't come from a particular place; they represent a range of genders and sexualities; they have very different spiritual lives and practices. But all of them share some key traits that you may consider in finding your kink-positive supporters:

>> People who love adventures.

>> People who are great listeners.

>> People who are working in sexuality education or health.

>> People who are fighting for justice in various arenas.

>> People whose only agenda for me is my happiness.

>> People who believe in my ability to create a life that suits me.

Another thing to consider when you're deciding who you want to share your excitement about kink with is finding people who are already in kinky relationships and the community. Consider the following:

>> Who in your life is the most kink-proficient and can help you get started?

>> Who might help connect you to other kinky people and community?

While preparing to come out, you may want to draw up your current *pod map*, which is a tool used to document your support system, or see who's there for you. (See Chapter 11 for information on pod mapping.)

These following types of questions can get you started:

>> Who are you closest to in your life right now?

>> Who takes care of you?

>> What practices are in place that support your joy and connection?

>> What events or art practices are most enlivening for you — think about sports, fandoms, cultural events, book clubs, and so on.

Getting out there: How to come out

As Jaime suggests in her book, *Great Sex: Mapping Your Desire*, when you're sharing information about your desire with friends or potential crushes, you can try to open up and enjoy yourself. Be playful! Sexphobia and anti-kink sentiment can create heavy burdens or fears when you're trying to share personal and intimate information. But you don't have to accept this overarching sex-negativity.

ACTIVITY

SHARING MY KINKS. You can decide how and when it's best for you to start getting out there and testing the kink waters. In this exercise, we provide our favorite ways to start thinking about how to come out.

1. **Write a four-line personal profile based on your newfound interest in kink.** Answer these types of questions:

    ● Who are you?

    ● What are you looking for?

    ● What forms of kink appeal most to you?

2. **Write a 90-second pitch about what you're looking for in terms of kinky play and kink life.** Answer these kinds of questions:

    ● Why does kink appeal to you?

    ● What are you excited about when you imagine your kink expression?

    ● What is most important for your friends or a crush to know about your interest in kink?

3. **Create a microblog post to describe your ideal kinky partnership.** For example, "I'm X; you're Y; they're Z; and we're XYZ together." If you're new to kink, your tweet might look like: *I'm a new kink explorer with romantic streak who loves to brat; you're a confident Dom and a disciplinarian with a tender heart; I'm looking for scene partners who live in the Midwest.* (See Appendix A for terms.)

4. **Create a vision statement for your desire.** A vision statement is a description of a future world that incorporates the transformational changes you aspire to. If you were fully living into your kinky aspirations, what would your life — socially, sexually, and in the day-to-day flows of family — look like?

    In my flourishing kink life, I have a submissive partner who is open to experimentation and to building kink community. We are discreet about who we are open with about our private life, but we also have a fantastic group of friends and playmates who enrich our social and intimate life together.

5. **Create a kink organizational chart that shows the kind of scenes and partnerships you are interested in.** Consider these kinds of questions:

    - Are you a monogamous kinkster? If so, what community connections, social groups, and kink training opportunities fill out your kink organization chart?

    - Are you looking for life partners or scene partners or both? What love flows and what kink flows do you envision? Where are these lines parallel and where do they intersect?

    - Do you envision a core partnership that serves as a hub with many lovers, scene partners, and friends that fan out as spokes on your wheel?

    - How do the kinksters in your life relate to each other?

This exercise is designed to get you to start to brainstorm and distill your thinking about kink and to place yourself at the center of your coming out and relationship-building process.

TIP

The information you generate here can help you open a conversation with a possible kink supporter, friend, or crush. Pull out that microblog, or share your new profile description, and start a free-flowing conversation. Find people who are delighted by your creative daring and ask them to create a counterpart to your discovery process so that you can start to find commonalities and exchange insights. In Chapter 13, you can find many more tips on where to go to start building relationships and community.

Planning when and where to come out

Selecting the right time and location to come out can greatly improve your outcomes. Here are some suggestions on when and where:

>> **In the great outdoors.** Spending time outside, taking a walk, getting some fresh air, or sitting in a quiet area are great places to have the chat. For example, "I asked you here because you're a person I trust, and I've discovered something important about myself that I want to share."

>> **During a coffee date.** Choosing to have this conversation while enjoying a cup of coffee or tea is a great idea. Select a table that's outside or not smashed up against others for a little privacy. Go during an off hour when the cafe may not be as busy. Sit facing each other. Ah, coffee. "Let me get your favorite."

>> **After an activity.** Coming out after spending time together doing something you both enjoy is another great option. Afterward you can share your exciting news in a quiet location.

>> **Over video or phone.** Coming out in person — the physical proximity, the ability to read body language, the option to hug, affirm, or comfort each other — is best.

However, meeting in person isn't always possible — for example, you live several hours apart — and in person may not be the best for you as a communicator (see Chapter 7 for a discussion about communication styles). If you can't have the conversation in person, the best-to-worst options are as follows:

- **Video.** Zoom, FaceTime, or other video messaging options allow you to make eye contact, read each other's body language, have an intimate conversation, and read tone and intent well.

- **Phone.** The phone lets your confidante hear your voice. They can tell when you're excited or taking a deep breath. You can take in when they're laughing or working hard to listen.

- **Text.** I don't recommend using text for high stakes conversations. People tend to talk in shorthand when texting. Tone is especially difficult to read: Is this person being sarcastic? Dismissive? Is the person joking *with* you or making a joke *of* you? People can also disappear mid-conversation. Texting has too many avenues for misinterpretation and misunderstanding.

- **Snail mail or e-mail.** I put these two options last because people seem to be using them less and less, especially snail mail. But writing a well-thought-out note about your process of learning about yourself, how you're thinking about the kinky life you want, and why you're confiding in this important person in your life can be a wonderful exercise. When Jaime works with clients, she often has them write letters they'll never send. Then over the next weeks or months, the content in these notes develops into a concrete process of disclosure.

  A well-constructed coming out letter gives the sender some physical space from the receiver, if that's what they need. And if the letter is well written, it can communicate a lot of complex ideas and hopes to the reader.

  Don't ever hit send on an e-mail when your blood pressure is up, your heart is beating fast, or you're mad at the person!

First, write your note with all the words that you think will express the kind of emotional space you're in. Then, you can work through your concerns to get to a final e-mail that feels centered and true. But in the end, you want to send a note that's measured — firmly grounded and abundantly who you are.

Avoiding hot-button places

Starting a coming out conversation at a major holiday dinner or in bed at the end of a long frantic day of work and/or managing kids is a recipe for disaster. And yet, in Jaime's practice as a sex coach, she can count many coming out conversations of all kinds that have happened in the following, very high stakes locales.

Here are places to steer clear of when having a coming out chat:

>> **In bed:** A disaster waiting to happen — don't do it! Couples often spill heavy relationship truths at 11 p.m. after an exhausting day in the place where they have had some of their most vulnerable, intimate moments together.

   If you're lucky enough to be sharing your bed with someone you lust for or love, respect the location of your intimacy and sex highlight reel. New crush confessions, coming outs, breaches of trust, major relationship changes — all these announcements need to be made in the light of day, fully hydrated, on neutral territory that won't be forever tainted by the possible pain and conflicts that might arise.

>> **In the car:** What is it about the car? So many big conversations happen in the car, but you can't make eye contact with the driver if the car is moving. Even if you can make and keep eye contact, you may feel trapped in the car if things start to go wrong.

   Nonetheless, a lot of coming out conversations happen on drives in the car. If you're going to do this, choose your confidante wisely. Don't wait until it's dark; consider the impact on the driver. Hydrate, snack, and choose a route where you know you can stop and take breaks.

Traveling the Long Road Together

Once you're out, discovering kink-positive friends is crucial for sustaining your kinky life. Of course, some people can't risk finding in-person kinky friends. But the good news is that you can create community in online spaces, groups, and meet-ups, even when you're relatively isolated in a hostile community or when you're navigating risks of social or economic retaliation (check out Appendix B for some resources).

As you approach kink life, here are a couple of ways you can create solidarity and reciprocity with the supportive pod you build:

>> **Choose friends because you're interested in them, not because they can do something for you or provide entree into a community.** Find people you want to build conversation and possibility with — people you want to support, as they support you, as you share resources, joy, and hardships over many years.

   Friends can lift you up and be proud of you. And when the going gets tough — job loss, breakups, parenthood demands, health crises, and so on — friends make all these changes survivable.

>> **Mind and tend to your pod.** There's so much uncertainty in today's world. Here's one thing that's entirely in your hands: your commitment to growing reciprocal, expansive, and joyful love among your friends. The universe often feels so big and full of dangers. You can't fix it all, but you can carry each other through.

Chapter **15**

Adapting Over Your Long Kinky Life

The novelist Octavia Butler notes in her landmark book, *Parable of the Sower* that *God is Change.* By that she means change is coming, and change is ever-present. While this may be true of *all* kinds of relationships, kink intimacies are a constant whirl of change, where needs are ever unfolding and even a single scene can shift and morph in unanticipated ways.

When you embrace rather than resist change, you greatly increase your chances of success in your kinky life.

In this chapter, you can find discussion of the life changes you may face while you age as a kinkster, including physical changes that impact your desire and capacity for various kink activities. Long-time kinksters often navigate diminishing libido, shifting expressions in your gender and sexuality, or are living with a disability. We also provide some stories from people who are making their way, over many decades, as kink practitioners through all the many changes that life brings.

Shifting Physical and Emotional Capacities

If you are fortunate to live a long life in kink, you'll observe and experience a lot of physical changes over time. As you age, your bodily capacity is in flux. If you have a kink passion that requires a particular kind of body strength — say, prolonged sessions of flogging your lover — you may have to adjust and find a different way to deliver on that particular lust. Or you may have to identify an entirely new set of practices that creates something unexpected or fresh for you both.

In kink life, this might mean that the specific space a relationship holds in your life may also shift. One scene partner might be a harsh Top, or loves to be caned, and now you aren't capable of being with them in the ways you were before. You may have been part of a monogamous kink couple for many years, and then as you lose certain capacities due to aging, you find that you want to recruit friends or crushes to help you deliver the experiences you and your partner are after.

When Jaime was a young kinkster for example, she needed really intense pain or domination to move into *subspace* (the intoxicated feeling of being high on a mix of hormones that are released by the intensity of kink play). The more sadistic the Top, the better. But as a parent in her 40s, her children's daily needs for intimacy and comfort took up so much time and energy, her body craved rest. Sadistic Tops didn't work for her at all then. Now, in her 60s, she has developed a praise kink; that is, she feels unmoored and vulnerable when her kink partners take extra notice of her in some way, showering her with affirmation. Fortunately, she has had a lot of different scene partners over the course of her kinky life, and also long-term partners who have been able to adjust and attend to her through these shifts.

If you enjoy your kinks over the long haul, you'll likely become skilled at discussing all kinds of lusts and kinky aspirations with your partners. Addressing your emotional and bodily changes due to aging will simply add another layer to these conversations.

This is a core underpinning of kink life, and often what attracts people to kink in the first place. It's the idea that desire and relationships change, and you can adjust and adapt to your partner's shifting needs and capacities as they emerge.

BODY CHANGES ARE REAL

Anna and I are really different than we were 15 years ago. For me, that's about a lot of changes in my body. I can't be in the same positions or hold the same body posture that I used to. My hands are curved and not as strong. So it's actually not as easy for me to do a lot of the things I used to do as her Top. I have to think about it, and it becomes like a puzzle, which is sometimes fun and sometimes really frustrating. **—Rox**

Coping with Libido Changes

As you experience the ups and downs of aging, so does your libido. It can be hard when your libido takes a nose-dive in the context of kink life. Your partner(s) may have to find new ways to support and care for you, while also getting their own needs met.

Grief is a natural response to a declining libido. But there's no need to panic. Staying curious about your changing relationship with lust and arousal can help you navigate these changes rather than deny them or shut down.

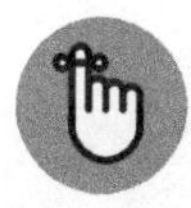

Willingness can be a starting point for sensual and sexual connection, rather than lust or attraction.

You can decide to maintain a kink relationship or set of practices because you value them, and you want them in your life, rather than feeling compelled by or driven by your libido as you have been in the past.

Another way to respond to a declining libido is to consider what other kinds of connections in your life are emerging as more important right now. Is your body directing you to prioritize other kinds of creativity or sensual experiences or intimacy?

Get curious, stay curious. The mysteries of aging always hold promise.

ACTIVITY

LIBIDO DETECTIVE. Ask yourself the following five questions to gain some insight into how you feel about the changes to your libido:

>> What's the hardest part about having a lower libido?

>> What relief or openings am I experiencing because my libido is less noisy or demanding?

>> What did my higher libido bring to my life that I miss?

>> How can I bring these things that I miss into my life?

>> What new or different intimacies can I bring into my life in the absence of being driven by my libido?

Just as your desires and abilities change over time, your answers to these questions may change over time, so you may need to revisit them for new insights in the future.

Living with a Disability in Kink Life

We live in a nation of increasingly aged and increasingly disabled people. The Centers for Disease Control notes that more than one in four people in the United States, or 28 percent of the population, is living with some kind of disability. If you are poor, BIPOC or queer, those numbers are even higher. In the 2023 National LGBTQ+ Women's Community Survey, 50 percent of respondents reported a mentally or physically disabling condition.

Disability can be a fact of life for many people, and yet systems of care have not seemed to catch up to this reality. The economic support net for disabled people and their families barely exists; the health care system is fragmented and expensive.

All of this means that disability is often a part of any person's intimate life. If you are kinky, the chance you will encounter disability among your partners often increases because many kinksters are connecting with multiple play partners.

In her landmark book, *The Future Is Disabled*, kink poet and disability justice activist Leah Lakshmi Piepzna-Samarasinha urges us to embrace that future:

> "It's radical to imagine that the future is disabled. Not just tentatively allowed to exist, not just *okay, I guess there's one white guy with a wheelchair, cool, diversity*. But a deeply disabled future: a future where disabled, deaf, mad, neurodivergent body-minds are both accepted without question as part of a vast spectrum of human and animal ways of existing, but where our cultures, knowledge, and communities shape the world . . . Have we ever imagined this, not just as a cautionary tale or a scary story, but as a dream?"

Piepzna-Samarasinha is encouraging you to throw off ableist fear and embrace changes to your body and your capacities. You can draw on the wisdom of your experience of disability and your disabled communities to chart new pathways toward intimacy.

Disposability culture says: disabled bodies are sexless and should be out of sight. Kink culture says: bring all of your complex self to the scene. You belong to yourself, first and foremost, and you and your kinky desires belong here.

REMEMBER

ALLOW FOR GRACE

I had a brain injury. That wasn't like a super sexy time. That wasn't a time that I had a lot of energy for other people because I had to spend so much energy just on my basic things. I could still do everything; it just took a lot more energy and my pain level was so high.

That also changed what I could engage in with my kink. So you know, like slaps across the face — even though that was something that I loved before my brain injury. But then it was like, *Oh no, my head*! My brain doesn't want to knock around like this right now. So, we have to take those things into consideration and allow each other grace. And then how do you figure out the boundaries or edges around those things? **—Anna**

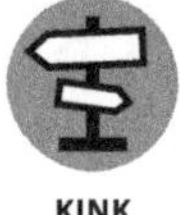

Body dysmorphia was a blessing. It drew me to everybody who was weird. This was Seattle in the early '90s and there was this burgeoning community of people who were living really different lives and converged with all of us living really different genders. So, I certainly saw kinky people who had really expansive ideas of how you walk in the world, and that was such a grounding for me. I was hanging with people who would like say — I'm a bulldagger, or I'm doing this art thing, or I'm . . . whatever. **—M'Bwende**

Dealing with Sexuality and Gender Shifts

Sharing your intimate life in kink community among such a resourceful and inventive group of players often has an impact on your sexual practices and your gender expression. It's possibly one of kink's greatest gifts — having opportunities to see greater depths and breadth in your own self-expression as you relate to outrageously different people. These simple observations suggest the positive impact kink play can have in growing different sides of yourself:

>> One scene partner is shy and reserved? This brings out your talky, protective side.

>> A kink crush has an inexhaustible libido? Now you're having more kink-plus-sex than you thought was even physically possible.

>> One scenester is more lustful when you wear short dresses and combat boots? Here comes your tough femme side.

>> A new play partner loves bondage? Now you're taking rope classes.

Jaime used to give a workshop called *Born This Way* to help participants tease out what parts of their sexual practices, gender expressions, and attractions were more fixed and what parts were more fluid or changing over time. We have re-created the experience in the following exercise.

MY DESIRE SPECTRUM. This exercise allows you to chart your interests around gender, sex, power, and kink. Using Figure 15-1, put an X in the circle where you land on the chart today. Put an X in different colors where you landed on the chart 5, 10, or 15 years ago. Put an aspirational red X on the chart where you wish to go.

My Gender

Feminine________________________Androgynous/Fluid________________________Masculine
○○

My Partner's Gender

Feminine________________________Androgynous/Fluid________________________Masculine
○○

Power/Agency in Sex

Penetrative________________________Versatile or Verse________________________Receptive
○○

Submissive________________________Mutuality/Mirroring________________________Dominant
○○

High Libido/frequency________________________Sex is good sometimes________________________No sex
○○

Kink Interests

Highly enjoy being hit________________________No hitting/impact Play
○○

Seek pain with pleasure________________________No Pain Play
○○

Tie me up/any bondage________________________No restraints
○○

I like it rough________________________I'm the tenderest flower
○○

Watch me/you have sex with others________________________Sex is just between us
○○

Sex in public (safety first!)________________________Sex is private
○○

Other Interests

Talk to me/tell me what you are doing________________________Silence is sexy
○○

Major kissing________________________Light kissing________________________No kissing
○○

Body worship/skinship________________________Cuddles!________________________No cuddling
○○

FIGURE 15-1:
Tracking Your
Desire Spectrum.

Sharing your desire spectrum with your scene partner(s) can be fun and revealing. If you're both (or all) curious about your sexual histories and where your kink practices land on your chart, sharing them can create a great story-sharing event full of laughter. It can reveal things you don't yet know about your partner(s) and create intimacy and possibility.

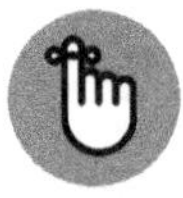

A great feature of aging is a tendency to have fewer f***s to give.

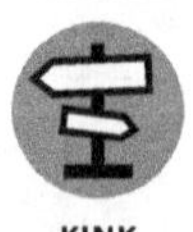

I think I'm more discerning as I get older. It's like if you can't check eight out of my ten boxes; I don't think so. When I was younger, I'd be: *Oh, you got three out of ten? Let s go. Let s do it!* Now, I'm like — don t even come close to me! **—Rox**

The Part of Tens

IN THIS PART . . .

Find a quick guide to the essentials of scene-making.

Identify the great kinksters throughout history from all over the world!

Discover amazing kinksters who are leading and thriving today!

Chapter **16**

Ten Hallmarks of a Vibrant Kink Sexuality

How will you know if your kinky sexuality is working for you? Simple! Your life will feel vibrant and full of possibility. You may experience challenges as you grow, and your needs may change. You may need to end some relationships and start others. Your social circle might expand or shift, but life is full of changes! A vibrant kink sexuality adapts, morphs, and pivots. And your self-esteem, joy, and intimate life grows alongside all of these changes.

In this chapter, you'll find ten characteristics of a healthy kink sexuality.

Your Process of Self-Discovery Is Never-Ending

You have made room for self-discovery and reflection, and it's paying off. Perhaps you've answered some of the many self-reflective questions in this book or tried the activities. Your journal is overflowing with new personal insights. You may have joined a social group or engaged a therapist to help you sift through some of this new material. Instead of feeling stuck and confused, you are on a path of life-long learning.

You're Acquiring Communication Skills and Kinky Tools

Understanding the particulars of your kinks is a new hobby for you. You're seeking out resources and events where you can acquire the skills essential to the kind of play you are passionate about. You're exchanging YES, NO, MAYBE lists (see Chapter 8), watching kink demonstrations, discovering ways to please yourself and your partners and take care of them. Instead of feeling isolated and incapable, you're trying out your new skills with like-minded people who are excited about your journey.

You Have at Least One Supportive Friend or Kink Confidante

When it comes to kink, what are the characteristics of a supportive friend? First and foremost – you've found someone whose only agenda is for you to find ways to pursue the kinky path of your dreams. Sometimes, a person who has been your closest confidante in other parts of your life is not the person who can accompany you on your kink discovery journey, and that's okay. It might be difficult for you to shift gears a bit around close friendships as you explore your kinks. You may need to recruit someone who is an experienced kink practitioner and suited to the task of supporting your needs as a questioning kinkster or a novice. As the saying goes, you can make new friends but keep the old.

You Have Found Kink Resources and Community

After doing some research and perhaps tenuously engaging with various events, you have found the right lanes for you kink exploration. You may or may not need in-person community connections, or you may or may not be particularly social. Whatever your personality — and your social, sexual, and kink needs — you have found engaging, supportive places to meet in person or online. You have people who get you and are interested and engaged in your process. You feel accompanied and appreciated.

You Can Go Through Changes Without Debilitating Distress

Some of your kink outreach is working and some isn't. You've been well received sometimes and rejected others. You've made some mistakes as you've tried different kinky practices and extended your trust. All of this is part of your experimentation and growth process. None of it is devastating because you've gained enough insight and self-confidence to have the bandwidth to try and fail, maybe several times. You have both the internal resources and enough external support in the form of friends or professional counsel to try new things and follow an imperfect path to a more authentic you.

You Have Clarity Around Your Boundaries

You'll use a safeword without hesitation, and you don't apologize for your needs. This practice may have taken some trial and error, but now you are safewording like a pro (see Appendix A). Your YES, NO, MAYBE list or your Kink Ten Commandments (see Chapter 8) state clearly where you are at in your kink discovery process.

You don't prioritize nice over honest. You understand that it's primarily your job to take care of yourself in a kink interaction, so your partners have the opportunity to be responsive and caring. You don't do things you don't want to do because you are trying to impress a crush or seduce a player.

You are getting to know yourself and speaking up for your needs on a deeper level, and that feels fantastic.

You're Experimenting with Your Kink Desires

You've come to clarity about the kind of kink connections you really want. You are pursuing them alone, online, or with people in person who are attractive to you on multiple levels. Most importantly, you're defining the right places for you to experiment. Your social group or online community is supportive; the people you are engaging with are trustworthy. This gives you the room to test the edges of your fantasies, or take on desires that have long been on your mind and in your fantasy life. Experimentation is fun! Finding out new things about your kink sexuality is amazing, an unparalleled gift.

You're Keeping Your Agreements

Among kinksters and non-kinksters, you are telling the truth and coming through on your commitments. You've become a reliable reporter of your wants and needs, and also your limits. You're not over-extending yourself — whether in the kinky scene, at home, or at work. Amazingly, growing your communication skills and kink practices is creating positive spill-over into your life beyond kink. Showing up in your scenes is helping you show up everywhere.

Your Life Is Working

Your involvement in kinky play isn't throwing everything else into chaos. While spending a lot of time reveling in the ecstatic rewards of kink play, you're still getting to work or class on time, taking care of your kids, paying your rent, doing your homework, and/or hanging out with your friends. You haven't disappeared from the rest of your life or abandoned your responsibilities. Kink play and relationships are adding to your universe, not disrupting or swallowing it.

You Feel Joyful, Curious, and Cherished Much of the Time

While struggling to open up about your kinks or find community has at times felt heavy, pursuing your true kink desires among people who care about you feels light and freeing. You may find yourself delving into vulnerable and emotionally painful territories in your kink practices, but you're taken care of in these relationships in ways you've never imagined possible. This brings an expansiveness to your life you didn't anticipate. It's spring in your heart, and a time of rebirth or reconnection in your body.

Chapter **17**

Ten Things to Help You Build Your Best Kinky Scenes

The most foundational step to building a kinky life is acknowledging your own desires (see more on this in Chapter 5). If you've already done a lot of work identifying what you want, you can pat yourself on the back because it's a profound step to have taken. This chapter provides ten more steps for your kink journey.

Fill Out a YES, NO, MAYBE List

YES, NO, MAYBE lists are useful for helping you-cut define what you're into, even if what you find out is something you never want to tell anybody. They can also be useful as a way of communicating with partners or potential partners. Sometimes the kink that brought you together with someone isn't the only thing you have in common, and these lists can tell you that.

As you read each entry on a YES-NO-MAYBE list (there's an extensive list in Chapter 8), you'll need to pay attention to which activities create the most powerful positive responses in you — which ones excite you, which ones you wish you could be doing right now.

You may also recognize there are options that you have powerful negative responses to. At this stage of your journey, what you're realizing is that these aren't things you want to do today, but many kinksters report that some of their favorite ways to play started out as things that scared or repulsed them, so it's worth paying attention over time.

Your YES-NO-MAYBE list offers a provocative snapshot. It's a temperature reading of where you are right now with your desires and your interests as you venture into kink.

Set Your Safeword

Safewords are a hallmark of kink culture. They are the magic declarations that provide an emergency brake to disrupt or end any kink scene. Whenever you start a new scene or play with someone for the first time, you'll need to work together to agree on a safeword. But you can also come up with one for yourself that you suggest by default when you're having that pre-scene discussion.

Even for kinksters who rarely use them, having an established safeword can give you a sense of power or control. Everyone involved in a scene has a personal tool to end it at any time, for any reason. Having an established safeword may create a touch point to remind you that your boundaries are important and only you can say where they are. You can read more about safewords in Chapter 8.

Get Online

Good news! Compared to the *olden days*, there's so much kink at your fingertips because of the Internet. If you aren't sure exactly what you want just yet, you can read erotic stories and see what most excites you. You can look up profiles on dating apps and see what other people are into. You can also get on social networking platforms and chat with other kinksters.

Fetlife (`https://fetlife.com`) is a major clearinghouse for kink where people of every gender, sexual orientation, and with any interests can find each other and even check out event listings. Dating apps can also provide the opportunity to make connections (see Appendix B for many options).

Even if you're not sure yet whether you want to meet anyone in real life (or if you're sure you don't), online spaces can provide an anonymous outlet for certain kinds of kink intimacy and can help you connect to yourself.

When connecting online, be as up front as you can about what you're looking for. A lot of people aren't looking for in-person play but many are. The more you can put in your profile about where you are in your journey, the easier it will be to attract people in a compatible situation or with similar interests.

Get Offline

You can build a totally fulfilling kink life entirely online or in the privacy of one-to-one connections with people you meet on the Internet. But if and when you're ready to step out, you can start looking for opportunities to connect to the kink community offline. Go to a munch (see Chapter 13), a class, or a play party. The biggest calendar of in-person events for kinksters in the U.S. is on Fetlife. Depending on where you live, local organizations and bars or clubs may also list events.

Enter a new social space as openly as you possibly can.

You may be showing up to a community that feels like it's already formed, where people already know each other. You may feel nervous about introducing yourself. On the other hand, you may also be put off by too much attention — by a rush to meet the newbie, which you may be! Just do your best to embrace the awkwardness — be friendly, be respectful. And if you find that you're really past your comfort zone, you can leave at any time. Paying attention to what works for you is great preparation for experimenting with kink.

In-person community can greatly expand and enhance your kink life. Many kinksters meet their spouses in these community spaces, form core friendships and extended families, and have tons of fun with people they might not have expected to click with when just looking at profiles online.

Find Your Location, Location, Location

Survey the options you have for where you can create the kink scenes you're starting to envision. Is there space in your home for what you want to do? What space is accessible and will make you feel most safe? Can your potential scene partners offer space? How well do you want to know someone before you're engaging in kink in their home, especially if you're doing anything where you will be bound or have your senses suppressed? Are there dungeons or clubs in your area? How far away would you have to go to get to one? Would you mind being in a semipublic setting? Would you love it?

Location options may change even if you stay in the same place for the rest of your life. Starting to survey your options and the kinds of spaces that would make you the most comfortable and excited will help you begin to create the life you want.

Volunteer

If you have discovered classes, parties, or other kink spaces, they often need volunteers. Giving your time and being of service to the community can give some kinksters a feeling of arousal and satisfaction in and of itself. But even if a service orientation isn't your kink, organizations and events producers love and appreciate volunteers to keep activities on track.

If you feel uncomfortable attending a play party as a relative newcomer or as an observer who isn't sure whether you actually want to play or not, having a volunteer role can help to calm you down and feel confident about what you're hoping to achieve in the space. It can give you a formal role for the evening. Volunteering also shows the people around you that you're serious about building community and that you're willing to put effort in.

Consider Equipment

Not every kink requires tools, but for those that do, watching demonstrations, making selections, and shopping for options are a big part of the fun. Do you like whips? Floggers? Paddles? Do you imagine yourself holding them or having them used on you? What do you imagine yourself wearing in a scene? Maybe nothing special or specific, or maybe clothes that help you dig into a role-play fantasy.

No matter where you are in your kink journey, your equipment can help fire your imagination, get your blood pumping, and support you as you think through what you want.

Make a Hydration Plan

Hydration often hinges on an event's set-up or location, but you may want to give some thought to how you're going to make sure you have access to water when you start to play. If you're playing in a dungeon or at a party, the hosts will probably have thought about this for you, but even if water is provided at a venue, you may want to bring your own water bottle so you definitely know where it is and that you can get to it if you need to.

Hydration may not be as sexy a consideration as thinking about what tools you want to bring to your dream scenes, but the stakes are similarly high. You need to make sure you've had or can have as much water as you need to go as long and hard as you plan.

Make an Aftercare Plan

Aftercare is any activity you need to pull yourself back together emotionally and physically after a scene. For many, you can best achieve this through loving, calming touch with your scene partners. But you know yourself and your needs better than anyone. You can start thinking about what may best serve you in that moment when play ends. Some people cuddle, others massage one another, and still others choose to chat about anything but kink in order to start the journey of reintegrating back to your daily life.

When you're actually post-scene and doing that integration work, you may find that the plans you made were all wrong for how you and your scene partner(s) actually feel. Stay open and talk as openly as you can about your shifting sense of the situation so that everyone can come down from your time spent together.

You can read more about aftercare in Chapter 9.

Keep an Open Mind

As you build your kinky life, there may be many twists and turns. You may find that you love doing things you never thought you would, and you may be surprised that long-term fantasies you've had that get you off every time when you're intimate with yourself just don't feel the same when they're acted out in person. You almost certainly will meet people who are deeply aroused by things that make you feel queasy or upset just to think about them.

REMEMBER

Try not to judge others — to yuck anyone else's yum — just as you would ask them not to judge or condemn you. Being as open as you can be toward the kinksters you meet on this journey will help you to stay open with yourself, build community, get your needs met, and lean into your most authentic kinky self.

Chapter **18**

Ten Kinksters in History

I f you've ever felt isolated in your kinky desires or made to feel like nobody else has wanted these same things, think again. History is full of people, including famous and accomplished people, who talked about, advocated for, and, above all, practiced their kinks.

Of course, the historical record can be hazy when it comes to matters of kink and sexuality, and certainly the kink lives of some people have been better documented than others. But as this list of kinksters born before World War II shows, kink has been a part of the human experience around the world and throughout history.

You may notice that some historical figures often held up as kinky pioneers, like the Marquis de Sade, are not listed here. This is because what de Sade was famous for was actually abuse, not kink. We've done our best to honor kink innovation and practice by excluding those who acted outside of the core kink values of consent and mutual respect.

Wolfgang Amadeus Mozart

Mozart was one of the most prolific and celebrated European music composers of the 18th century. Originally from Salzburg, Germany, Mozart became skilled in piano and violin and began to compose music by the age of five. Before he died, he had written over 800 pieces of music that crossed classical genres.

In terms of kink, Mozart's surviving letters detail his interest in analingus (see Appendix A), farts, and even suggest experience with scat play. This theme is visible in some of his compositions, like the song, "Leck mich im Arsch," which translates to "lick me in the a**."

James Joyce

Another historical figure who was fixated on farts was celebrated Irish author, James Joyce. Joyce was born at the end of the 1800s in Dublin. Joyce authored some of the most noted English-language literature of his day, including *A Portrait of the Artist as a Young Man*, *Finnegans Wake*, and *The Dubliners*. His novel, *Ulysses*, was at the heart of a legal controversy having originally been banned under obscenity law because of his metaphorical description of sexual acts.

Joyce wrote extensively about his personal interest in the farts of women. He enjoyed incidental farts but also professed his desire for women to fart on his face. It seems he also enjoyed his own farts, particularly when directed at his female partners.

Seiu Ito (伊藤晴雨)

Seiu Ito was born around the same time as James Joyce, but on the other side of the world in Tokyo, Japan. He showed an interest in the arts from a young age. As the son of a metalworker, he learned sculpture, spent time studying Japanese stagecraft, pored over woodblock prints, and became a highly skilled painter.

Seiu Ito is considered to be the father of modern Japanese rope bondage. Ito called the practice *kinbaku* (緊縛), which literally translates as "tight binding," and enjoyed the art as both sexual performance and artistic inspiration. He took torture practices from Japanese history and reconfigured them in ways that appealed to his kinky sensibility, tying up consenting models, taking photographs, and then painting based on the photos. His paintings became so popular around Japan that the practice of rope bondage also flourished and has been passed down to contemporary kinksters the world over.

Theresa Berkley

Theresa Berkley was a 19th-century English Dominatrix who ran a famous brothel in London. Berkley was known as a "governess," which was a particular kind of Dom woman that referenced the kind of discipline used by tutors and nannies. She enjoyed switching to a certain extent, but clearly preferred the Dominant role, working with clients of all genders, many of whom were from the English aristocracy.

Berkley specialized in various form of bondage and impact play, enjoying tools such as whips, leather straps, and hooks and pullies. She even used plants such as holly brushes that held specific symbolic weight because it was the kind of tool an actual governess may have used for discipline in the period. Berkley is remembered for her innovations in bondage equipment, including the kinds of apparatuses she would tie clients and partner to for scenes. Some of these can still be found in use today.

Jean-Jacques Rousseau

If you've ever taken a political philosophy class, you may have read the writings of Jean-Jacques Rousseau, born in 1712 in what is now Switzerland. Rousseau spent his life seeking to understand human inequality, and ultimately assigning its source to the concept of private property. He was greatly interested in the ways people might create political systems that respect the freedoms of individuals while also serving the group as a whole.

Philosophy, though, was not the only area of his life where he showed an interest in power and inequality. Rousseau was a submissive with a taste for being demeaned, and spanked by women. He was an innovator as a memoirist, where he offered self-reflection on his kinks with lines like, "To be at the knees of an imperious mistress, to obey her orders, to have to beg her pardon, have been for me the sweetest delights."

María Getrudis Arévalo

In 1797, the Catholic Holy Office in Mexico opened an investigation against María Getrudis Arévalo for engaging in sexual acts they saw as sacrilegious. These records offer an imperfect but vivid look into the kink life of an impoverished Latin American woman at the turn of the 18th century.

She was accused of masturbation with holy objects, including stimulating herself with crucifixes and spreading her menstrual blood across icons as a part of her erotic rituals. What authorities saw as most damning was when she began to hide undigested holy communion in her mouth and smuggle it out of mass to be taken home and used in masturbation.

Betty Paërl

Born in the Netherlands in 1935, Betty Paërl was many things in her life — a trans woman, a mathematician, an anarchist, an anti-colonial activist, and a professional Dom. After earning her PhD in Mathematics, Betty became active in the protest movement in solidarity with the Dutch colony of Suriname in South America, which was seeking independence.

Throughout her life, she advocated for open discussion of sexuality, including how kink can be a space for trans people to explore gender and find their way to their truest selves. She explored many facets of kink, but found particular satisfaction as a Dom, experiencing gender euphoria in the respect she was given when she wielded the whip while embodying femme power. When she was fired from her university job for her identity and activism, she spent much of the rest of her life doing sex work and writing about math and politics.

Queen Nzinga of Ndongo and Matamba

Queen Nzinga was a southwest African monarch from the 16th and 17th centuries who ruled over territory that is now a part of Angola. She is noted for her skills as a military tactician and negotiator who fended off encroachment from the Portuguese empire during the development of the Atlantic slave trade.

She was also famous for her sexuality, having had numerous male lovers. Of course, it's important to question historical sources written by white men who were speaking about the sexuality of a Black African woman monarch, a dynamic that may give us a warped image of her. It's possible, or even likely, that some European writers may have exaggerated the degree to which she was a brutal Dom in her sex life in order to cast her in a negative light, but, if nothing else, it seems clear that Queen Nzinga had a kink for group sex and often favored the strongest men in her community.

Empress Wu Zetian (武則天)

In over two thousand years of dynastic Chinese history, only one woman ascended to the throne in her own right. Her name was Wu Zetian and her rule lasted from the years 624 to 705. She began her career in the palace by occupying the throne on behalf of her husband and then later her son, before dispensing with these backdoors to power and taking control herself. Among her royal achievements were reviving the Chinese economy and rooting out corruption in the royal court.

Similar to Queen Nzinga, she was remembered by many as being a dominant woman in the context of sex as well as politics. But it can be difficult to discern, over a thousand years later, whether she was really a kinkster or if these were rumors intended to harm her reputation and prevent the rise of other women to positions of power. It does seem that she ran her sex life the way she ran other parts of her life, disregarding what her community considered appropriate for women, like having multiple lovers, stating her desires outright, and performing sex acts that nobody else would.

Enheduanna

The final figure on our list was a princess and priestess in the world's first city, Uruk, around the year 2300 BCE. She was the daughter of King Sargon the Great and the high priestess of the goddess Inanna, whom many consider to be a kind of Dominatrix deity. Enheduanna is universally revered in archeology for her contributions to history and literature using the *cuneiform alphabet,* one of the world's oldest writing systems. In fact, she is considered the earliest named author in history.

The rituals of Enheduanna involved many practices that are recognizable to kinksters today, like flagellation, discipline, and all kinds of pain play. Worshippers also played with gender, with men being feminized for short scenes and trans women undergoing ceremonies for gender transformation after which they lived as priestesses. Of course, it's difficult to be certain that these religious practices were kinks in the modern sense, but it shows that rituals involving bondage, agony, and discipline are as old as human civilization itself.

Chapter **19**

Ten (or so) Contemporary Kink Trailblazers

Every day, kinksters are creating new ways of being, trailblazing ideas and practices of sexuality, intimacy, and community. In this chapter, you'll find a list of thinkers and doers from all over the world who have publicly claimed their kinks and extolled their practices and communities so that we have more space to be ourselves and revel in our kinky joys.

Midori (美登里)

Midori (1966–) is a Japanese-German-American author, advocate, and teacher on sex. Born in Kyoto, she moved to the U.S. when she was 14, positioning her to foster an exchange of ideas around kink, art, and beyond.

Midori is the founder of Rope Dojo and *ForteFemme: Women's Dominance Intensive*. She is noted for writing the first English language book on Japanese rope-play, the now classic *Seductive Art of Japanese Bondage*. Midori has worked extensively with therapists, educators, and coaches to develop cultural competence in serving kinksters. Her ethos of self-actualization, shame reduction, and justice within the world of kink, can be encapsulated by her quote, "By dominating someone, you may be able to help someone else free themselves to be themselves."

Guy Baldwin

In the early '80s, Guy Baldwin (1946–) broke ground by asserting that kinksters aren't sick. As a Leatherman and a psychotherapist, Baldwin's organizing built on the declassification of homosexuality as a mental illness. He has spent a lifetime creating a world where kinky people can access mental health support without being stigmatized. He also started the first database of mental health professionals who were supportive in the areas of kink and polyamory.

Baldwin has held two Leather contest titles — Mr. National Leather Association and International Mr. Leather. For many years, he published fiction and nonfiction including a much beloved monthly column in *Drummer* magazine, which was ultimately compiled into *Ties that Bind*.

Li Yinhe (李银河)

Li Yinhe (1952–) is a sexologist, activist, and the first person in China to get a PhD in the Sociology of Gender. Her work has included translations of key foreign works on sex, as well as research on sexuality in Chinese history and literature, like the kinky classic *The Plum in the Golden Vase* (金瓶梅).

She has advocated for a Chinese sexual revolution that she believes must bridge the divide between rural and urban and include the legalization of group sex, pornography, and sex work. A self-identified heterosexual, Dr. Yinhe has also worked to push the Chinese government to guarantee the rights of LGBTQ+ people to work and marry, free from discrimination.

Mollena Williams-Haas

If you've ever seen *The Wiz*, you've heard the voice of Mollena Williams-Haas (1969–) because she sang backup to Lena Horne on the "Believe in Yourself" reprise for the 1978 movie. Since then, she's worked on films like *Skin & Bone* from 1996 and 2012's *IMPACT*.

Williams-Haas has also written extensively about kink. Her most famous essays include "Tables Briefly Turned" and "On Collars and Closure and Owning Myself." But her most noted contribution came in "BDSM and Race Play," in which she offers the perspective of a Black woman thinking critically about race and kink in the collection, *Best Sex Writing 2010*.

Dorothy Allison

Dorothy Allison (1949–2024) was a giant in the world of lesbian literature and sex organizing. Her astonishing novel on child sexual abuse, *Bastard Out of Carolina* was a finalist for the National Book Award in 1992, making her the first lesbian to ever make the list.

But prior to this singular achievement, Allison was fired from her job at *Poets and Writer's* magazine in 1982 for her pro-kink arguments at the landmark Barnard Sex Conference. This intellectual and activist clash launched the Lesbian Sex Wars, wherein one wing of the community adopted an anti-porn organizing strategy that equated porn and kink with violence against women. While the other — with Allison's organization NYC's Lesbian Sex Mafia in the lead — argued that the right to engage in kink was a sexual liberation struggle that lesbians must take up. For nearly a decade Allison and her peers in LSM were vilified, and then the genius of *Bastard Out of Carolina* catapulted pro-sex organizing to much more serious footing among lesbians and all feminists.

Ignacio Hutía Xeiti Rivera

Ignacio Rivera (1971–) is a queer, Boricua, Taíno activist, performer, and cultural sociologist who embraces sexual liberation as a vehicle for ending racial and sexual violence. In the '90s, Ignacio broke ground by organizing BIPOC play parties out of their apartment in Brooklyn. At the time, according to Rivera, kink and polyamory were seen "as a white thing." And play spaces were often prohibitively costly and white-dominated. As a founding board member of Queers for Economic Justice, Ignacio threaded together political analyses on economic, racial, and sexual justice in their work.

For more than 25 years, Ignacio has created comprehensive sex education writing and workshops, original plays and performance art, and queer and trans centric kink porn, touring the country at major universities and community centers. Their biographical film, *They*, was among the first film projects to articulate and explore nonbinary BIPOC identity. Currently co-director of the *Heal Sweet Home Project*, Ignacio draws on abolitionist practices to end child sexual abuse.

Carol Queen

In 2009, Carol Queen (1957–) was invited to Oxford University to debate the idea that promiscuity is a virtue, not a vice. This position perhaps best encapsulates her life's work in the trenches for kink. Queen describes herself as a sex-positive feminist, often using porn to educate as well as stimulate. Through her *Bend Over Boyfriend* series, she's opened up the world of pegging for many, and in her tutorial, *Exhibitionism for the Shy: Show Off, Dress Up and Talk Hot*, she explores and demystifies many of the worlds of kink, including voyeurism, exhibitionism, and role-play.

Queen was the founder of San Francisco's Center for Sex and Culture, a space that provided "judgment-free education, cultural events, a library/media archive, and other resources to audiences across the sexual and gender spectrum" until the space was lost to the city's aggressive gentrification. Queen has served as resident sexologist and historian for the trailblazing women-owned Good Vibrations sex toy shop.

Susie Bright

When remembering the Lesbian Sex Wars (see Dorothy Allison earlier in this chapter), one of the key warriors on the side of kink was Susie Bright (1958–). She co-founded and edited the first women-produced sex-magazine, *On Our Backs*, from 1984 to 1991. Susie wrote an advice column called "Susie Sexpert," refining a voice that would go on to be among those defining discourse on lesbian sexuality for years to come. Bright was also a member of the collective that created Good Vibrations, a groundbreaking feminist sex store in San Francisco.

Susie has been active across many social justice movements, including for labor rights and anti-war. As a young person, she was active with an underground newspaper called, *The Red Tide*, and became a plaintiff in a successful case to sue the Los Angeles Board of Education for the rights of minors to be able to publish their ideas without school censorship.

Selogadi Mampane

Selogadi Mampane is a teacher and advocate for inclusive education in South Africa. She has specialized in the needs of students with disabilities.

Selogadi is also a performance artist and an advocate for sexual liberation. When she was crowned Ms. South Africa Leather in 2015, she became the first Black woman in Africa to be a formal Leather title holder. A performance artist and activist from Tshwane, Selogadi went on to represent at the International Ms. Leather in San Jose, California where she placed second.

Eric Rofes

Eric Rofes (1954–2006) was a proud gay man and a kink activist who married the messages of LGBTQ+ liberation, sexual freedom, and the fight against HIV. He was part of a young "gay mafia" that founded *Gay Community News* in Boston in the '70s, and eventually served on the board of the National LGBTQ Task Force and as executive director of the Los Angeles LGBT Center and San Francisco's AIDS Service Organization, SHANTI.

As a kinkster, Rofes was critical of abstinence-only sex education and HIV prevention efforts that closed gay bathhouses and stigmatized sex. He wrote treatises on gay male culture and resistance to sexism, homophobia, and anti-kink biases in the fight against AIDS. Rofes authored 13 books including *Reviving the Tribe* and *Dry Bones Breathe*, where he insisted on the meaning of queer and kink desire: "We value the enactment of our desires and will not always give them up in a grand gesture of sacrifice to the AIDS epidemic." Eric believed in community-based education and founded the *Gay Men's Health Leadership Academies* to train those working on HIV advocacy about what a sexual liberation-centric approach could look like.

Tyler McCormick

When Tyler McCormick won International Mr. Leather in 2010, he made history. That year, he become the first trans man, the first person who uses a wheelchair, and the first person from New Mexico to take home the most prestigious Leather title in the United States.

Tyler has used his platform to speak to the old guard Leather community and open minds about what true accessibility and trans belonging could look like in kink spaces. During his title year, he noted that his very presence meant that people were paying more attention to accessibility.

V. M. Johnson

V. M. Johnson (1950–) says she came into kink when she was bitten by a vampire at the age of 17 and was given vampire blood back. Active in the Leather lesbian scene since the '70s, Johnson has been the head judge for Ms. World Leather and many other Leather contests across the continent.

She has been passionately involved with preserving the history of the kink communities. She has worked with the Leather Archives & Museum, as the well as being the director and senior griot of the Carter/Johnson Library and Collection, a traveling kink library and archive. She is the author of two books, *Dhampir: Child of the Blood* and *To Love, to Obey, to Serve: Diary of an Old Guard Slave*. And in 2012, she became the first woman and the first Black woman to receive the National LGBTQ Task Force's Leather Leadership Award.

Naria Lei B. Jordan

Naria Lei B. Jordan is a longtime sex radical and the co-owner of DESIRE 2.0, a queer women's kink production company. Naria has been active in the queer/kink community for over 42 years as a practitioner, organizer, activist, and educator in the Leather High Kinky Arts. Identifying as genderqueer, he has held the titles of Ms. San Diego Leather 2002 and Southern California Leather Woman 2012–2013. His leadership has included service to The Leather Realm San Diego, South Bay Pride, International Ms. Leather and Boot Black, and the National LGBTQ Task Force.

Naria co-founded two women's-only leather groups in Washington, DC — Lesborados and S/Mazons — and was a founding editor and writer for the groundbreaking collective publication *Black Leather . . . In Color*. He also facilitated the Women's BDSM Rap in San Diego and co-facilitated the Women's BDSM Forum in California's Central Valley.

Appendix **A**
Glossary

Kink For Dummies is a book about kink desire and relationships among consenting adults, and the ways they relate intimately and sexually. Many of the terms in this book clearly delineate sexual practices, experiences, and characteristics. Please proceed accordingly.

Accountability: Taking responsibility for your choices and the impact of those choices on others. While a lot of accountability talk centers on getting someone else to be accountable for perceived wrongs, accountability work starts with the self.

Activated or activation: The state of being launched into a fight, flight, freeze, or fawn response. A synonym for triggered.

Adrenaline, cortisol, and endorphins: Hormones that can be released in the brain and other parts of the nervous system during kink play that reduce pain and increase happiness.

Aftercare: The set of activities that close a kink scene wherein partners re-integrate into common society. Hydration, connection, and attending to everyone's needs are the cornerstones of aftercare.

Age gap play: Playing with the taboo of an older partner "seducing" or manipulating a younger, inexperienced partner.

Age play: Playing with self-expression in various ages and stages. A lot of age play involves taking on infant or toddler states of being and having a partner care for you.

Alchemy of desire: When you throw all of your yearning into the fire of lust and connection, something new and unexpected gets made.

Analingus: Oral sex, such as licking or sucking, on the anus.

Anal fisting: Penetration of the anus with a hand and sometimes wrist or forearm.

Anal teasing: Some kinksters like to play at anal penetration as a way of exciting or winding up their partners or pushing on their fears.

Anal toys/plugging: Anal plugs are a much beloved sex toy and can be used for stretching the anus in preparation for penetration by a partner, or one can plug a partner as "punishment" or as a way to control, or to pleasure via a remote-control vibrator, or to secure ejaculate inside.

Anti-sex or sex-negative culture: Cultural beliefs that sex is dirty, wrong, dangerous, or scary and that it's necessary to strictly control and severely limit sexual expression and practices. As an opposite, sex-positive beliefs regard sex as sacred, healing, beautiful, and/or a pleasurable way to connect.

Asexual or ace: Asexuals, often self-described as Aces, generally do not experience sexual desire. Nonetheless, Aces report attractions and a yearning for intimacy based on other facets of connection. In this vein, many Aces pursue intimacy via their kink desires.

A worship:** A kink focused on reverent attention to the a**.

Bags: Any kind of full-body restraint used for bondage. Body bags, also known as sleep sacks, can enclose a person from their toes to either the neck or even over the head.

Beating: Hitting a scene partner or lover consensually, for pleasure.

Begging: Submitting or groveling to a Dom or scene partner for pleasure.

BIPOC: An acronym for Black, Indigenous, and other People of Color meant to emphasize the primacy of the genocide of Indigenous people and enslavement of Black people as foundational to the formation racism and racial identity the U.S.

Body slapping: Open-handed hitting of the body for pleasure.

Bodyworkers: Healers who work with the body such as massage therapists.

Bondage: Activities that restrict the movement of your partner for their pleasure.

Bootblack: A revered tradition in Leather communities wherein the kinkster provides careful, submissive care of leather boots or other treasured leather gear. During revered Leather competitions worldwide, a major award goes to the best bootblack, who performs their skills for the crowd.

Bottom: Bottom has two meanings in the kink world. Sometimes it is used as a synonym for sub or submissive in a Dom/sub pairing. When it comes to penetrative sex, it can also mean the partner being penetrated. These two meanings may not always line up. For example, a bottom (the partner being penetrated) could be the Dom in charge of the scene.

Boy nextdoor/girl nextdoor: A kink that draws on the romcom trope of having a formative crush on your next-door neighbor.

Bratting: Mouthing off to a Dom or scene partner to elicit a disciplinary response.

Breast torture: Pain-inducing binding of the breasts for pleasure.

Breath play: Restricting the airway passage of a lover or scene partner for pleasure. Breath play requires safety training so that the person initiating it has a clear understanding of the physiology of breath restriction and safe neck holds.

Cages: Kinksters who love bondage or restraint may choose to be locked in a cage by a trusted partner for pleasure. Limiting movement can be the operative kink here, or surrendering power.

Caning: Smacking a scene partner or lover on the a** or legs are the most common forms of caning. Caning delivers a specific visceral experience, unique sounds, and pain, sought after by sadists and masochists alike.

The Carnal Prayer Mat (肉蒲團): A 17th century Chinese erotic novel that details the period's sexual practices, including kink practices, and how they intersect with Chinese religion and spirituality.

Clit fingering: Playing with the clitoris with one's fingers. A highly lauded source of pleasure among those possessed of a clitoris.

Clothed/naked scene: A kink dynamic where one partner is clothed and the other is stripped bare. It is often abbreviated according to the gender of those involved. For example, CFNM stands for "clothed female, naked male," or CMNM for "clothed male, naked male."

Clothes pins/zip strips: Use of any rigid, pre-formed contraction joint in kink play. These restrict blood flow to the area clipped or pinned and create a rush of pain/pleasure upon release.

Coming out: Sharing one's identity, desire, fantasy, or set of private practices with another to create community or a stronger sense of self. Some kinksters may choose to come out broadly, or publicly. Many do not.

Consensual non-consent/rape play: Role-play during which rape is simulated, often through careful co-creation of the scene in advance. May also involve pre-consenting to a Dom that the role-play can take place unexpectedly.

Consent or scene container: The agreements that all kinksters involved in a scene make to ensure there's a shared understanding of when play starts, what the limits are, and how to signal an all-stop or end to the scene if needed.

Contract: A formal, written set of agreements co-created by kinksters — often a Dominant/submissive (or Top/bottom) — that clearly outlines the rules of engagement for kink play. Some contracts create the basis for 24/7 kink dynamics in the relationship (see Chapter 4).

Corporal Punishment: Corporal punishment, literally meaning punishment of the body, has an iconic place in kink culture referencing school-based corporal punishments such as smacking the hands with ruler and caning. On the home front, spanking children is a long-held practice that persists in some parenting cultures and holds significant space in the kink imagination.

Cosplay: The term cosplay originated in Japanese fandoms to mean dressing up as a character from an anime, manga, video game, or novel. A combination of the words "costume" and "play."

Cuckolding: Classic cuckolding involves a husband offering his wife to another man for sex and then watching that sex from the sidelines, for a pleasurable experience of emasculation or humiliation. People of all genders, sexualities, and relationship forms play with cuckolding.

Cuffs: A common form of restraint, cuffs are most often fastened to the wrists or the ankles.

Cutting: Using razor blades in any form of play, alone or with others.

Daddy and Mommy play: a person of any gender or sexual orientation may take on a fatherly, motherly, or otherwise paternal role with their kink partners. Daddy or Mommy play is most often directive, corrective, or babying.

Deep throating: involves taking a penetrative object, often a penis or dildo, into the deep recesses of the throat while engaging in a blow job. Many kinksters find deep throating highly gratifying around their need to dominate or submit.

Desire Mapping or desire inventory: A process of individual or collective inquiry that uncovers a person's stories about sex and longing for the purpose of discovering one's truth and pursuing intimacy and joy.

Devastation play: A set of kinky practices that draw on fantasy re-enactment of historic devastation or present-day abuses such as rape, enslavement, biases against certain religions, genders, races, or other groups, and colonial displacement — for pleasure. Devastation play can be transformative, and also emotionally risky or devastating, for kinksters with a family history of surviving these abuses.

Dildo: Any oblong object used for stimulating yourself or a partner through insertion; can be strapped onto the body of the penetrator or manipulated by hand.

DILF: Acronym for Dad or Daddy I Would Love to F*ck, which could apply to the pursuit of any older man or masculine presenting person.

Discipline: Using rules and punishment as a form of kink play for pleasure.

Disposability Culture: Cultural mind-set that prioritizes judging and excising or exiling people in your life rather than working to address, repair, and extend the life of relationships.

Dom (Dominant): Descriptor of a person of any gender or sexual orientation who is gratified by demonstrating aggressive, directive, and/or controlling behaviors to the delight of a consenting partner.

Domination: Taking power in a kink exchange.

Dominatrix: A woman or femme who takes the dominant role in a kink scene or dynamic (see Chapter 4), sometimes as a profession.

Double penetration: Being penetrated by more than one person or object simultaneously, sometimes in the same orifice or opening.

Dungeon: A kink space, often set up with furniture, implements, and supportive gear for kink play. Can be a public shared space, often run as a business or club, or can refer to a private space.

Edging: A practice of repeatedly approaching orgasm but backing off each time in order to prolong the experience, either for yourself or for a partner.

Edge play: Play among kinksters wherein they intentionally approach one or more of the players' boundaries. This can also refer to playing with edging, see previous.

Electrostimulation: Kink use of transcutaneous electrical nerve stimulation (TENS) device for pleasure.

Endorphin Rush: A surge in the release of endorphins, a morphine-like chemical in the brain that triggers pleasure and pain relief.

Enslavement play: Kink play that plays with ownership or total control of one or more partners, sometimes including references to historical practices of slavery.

Exhibitionism: A kink for revealing or displaying your body, particularly parts of the body that cultural norms deem inappropriate for others to see.

Face-sitting: When one person sits on another person's mouth or on their face, forcing the other person to give up a degree of control while administering cunnilingus, analingus, or a blow-job.

Facial: When one partner ejaculates on another's face. Often associated with semen, may also describe ejaculatory fluid from a woman's urethra.

Fake public use: Pretending that you or your sub are for spontaneous public use (see definition) while playing out a pre-choreographed scenario.

Fan fiction: Smutty, romantic, or cute stories that use real people like celebrities or fictional characters as their base for world-building and playing out sexy or kink scenarios.

Fantasy: In terms of kink, any sexy situation you can imagine or storyline that expands your kink or sexual imagination and amplifies your arousal.

Femme: Femme is an umbrella term to mean feminine people regardless of whether they identify as men, women, or nonbinary people.

Fetish: A synonym for a kink, anything that intensifies a person's arousal.

Fetishwear: Encompasses a wide world of gear and clothing related to people's kinks. For many, it calls to mind styles associated with roles like dominatrices or communities like Leather men, but events where the dress code calls for fetishwear could include people in a wide range of outfits from Furries to rubber diving suits to yoga pants.

Fingering: Using the fingers in sex, often specifically used for stimulation of the clitoris or anus with fingers.

Finger f*cking: Sexual penetration with fingers.

Fisting: Penetrative sexual play that involves inserting a closed fist into the vagina or anus of your partner.

Flogging: Kink play in which the sub is struck repeatedly with an implement made of many strips of fabric, often leather.

Foot fetish: Heightened or obsessive devotion to the feet is a popular kink, including observing, massaging, adorning, worshiping, or using them in sex.

Forced dressing: A Dom may consensually command a sub to wear an item or particular style of clothing as a form of humiliation or control of their partner's pleasure.

Forced feminization: Any set of activities that moves a masculine assigned or identified person into feminine role or space, as demanded by a Dom.

Forced orgasm: Kink play in which a scene partner pushes the person submitting over the edge, into orgasm.

Formal clothing: Play while wearing formal clothing to control or arouse a partner. This can cross over with Gender Play because formal clothing can be highly gendered. For example, it can include playing with the symbolic power of a tuxedo or a ballgown.

Fkbuddies/Friends with Benefits:** Someone, possibly someone you are friends with, whom you have sex with without a romantic attachment or an agenda for a more committed relationship.

Furry: A kinkster who enjoys creating animal characters with human characteristics. Furries may dress up as these characters in kink play.

Gags: A kink tool to restrict a sub's ability to speak or make noise with their mouths.

Gangbang: A group sex scene in which there are multiple penetrators focused on one person who is being penetrated.

Geeking out: Excitedly going deep into research or discussion of a topic that interests someone.

Gender play: Gender play involves using the symbols of masculinity and femininity in kink. It could mean inhabiting a gender that a kinkster doesn't identify with in their daily lives or being pushed by a play partner to act in a gendered way that elicits a reaction or heightens their arousal.

Genital torture: Hurting or verbally degrading a person's genitals.

Genital worship: Highly praising or lovingly attending a person's genitals.

Glory hole: A hole in a wall or sheet through which sex can take place without the participants seeing each other's faces.

Governess: A codeword and particular type of dominatrix in the 19th century that used the symbols of a stern, punishing private tutor.

Hentai (ヘンタイ): Erotic Japanese animation and comics.

Hotwifing: A kink wherein a husband or Dom partner of any gender allows someone else to have sex with the sub partner, or *hot wife*, and feels pride and arousal from the sharing. Hotwifing is in the family of cuckolding play.

Hot wax: Use of hot wax in kink play to cause intense sensations on the skin.

Human auctioning/appraisal: Role-play in which the sub's value is assessed and then they are sold at auction, often with reference to historical slave auctions. Auctions are part of the arena of devastation play.

Human furniture: if you like providing your lap to a Top for their pleasure, or if you imagine getting on all fours and offering your back as a seat to a stranger or play partner, you may be interested in serving as human furniture in your kink life.

Humiliation: Being shamed and having your vulnerabilities exposed, publicly or privately, often result in feelings of humiliation. Some kinksters gratified by feeling humiliated by their Dom or Top.

Hypnotism: The practice of consensually putting someone into a trance-like state in which they are more open to suggestion and control, in the context of kink play.

Impact Play: Kink play involving one or more partners striking other partners with their hands or other tools.

Incest play: Fantasy role-play involving sex with members of your imaginary immediate family or primary caregivers.

Interrogation: A scene in which a Dom systematically questions a sub, sometimes drawing on questioning tactics used by the military or police.

Kidnapping: Consensually abducting someone and holding them "against their will," conducted as kink role-play but perhaps done without the sub's prior knowledge of when and where it will take place.

Kink: A kink is any intimate or sexual activity that registers as outside of the "norm" and greatly amplifies one's experience of vulnerability and arousal.

Kinksters: People who love and revel in their unconventional or intense desires — also known as kinks — are kinksters.

Latex: A kink for the material of latex rubber, often wearing it as compressing garments.

Leather: A kink that reveres or even worships the smell, look, and feel of leather. Also a kink sub-culture based around a leather-centric aesthetic presentation, as well as a set of membership clubs, bars, pageant-like contests, and practices such as the creation of Leather families.

Leather contest: Based loosely on beauty pageants, Leather contests allow kinksters to show off their looks, fashion, and skills in a competitive context that often also raises money for HIV care or other health or community-building work.

Leather family: A familial structure within Leather culture in which people integrate their kink or Leather dynamics and relationships into their chosen family structures. Often but not always includes strong hierarchies.

Lesbian Sex Wars: A collective debate in the 1970s and 1980s among lesbian feminists about whether kink and pornography were inherently violent and anti-woman. A pro-sex wing of the women's and queer movements emerged from this debate that thrives on today.

LGBTQ+: Acronym for the community of lesbians, gay men, bisexuals, transgender people, and queers.

Libido: One's desire for intimate or sexual connection, commonly discussed as *sex drive,* but many people who don't pursue sex with others have robust libidos. Libido fluctuates wildly among people and across the lifespan.

Marking: Leaving permanent or impermanent marks on a partner's body for pleasure or to signal ownership.

Master: A designation for a Dom that suggests total control, and may or may not reference playing out a Master/slave dynamic.

Medical: Role-play in which one or more partners takes on the character of a doctor, nurse, or other medical professional, and the other plays the patient.

MILF: Acronym for Mom or Mommy I Would Love to F*ck, which could apply to the pursuit of any older woman or femme-presenting person. Like DILF, MILF is a highly sought-after kink scenario.

Military: Military scenes or military play use the symbols of armed forces, weaponry, and their violent power in a kink context.

Monster/beast: Role-play in which one or more partners takes on a monstrous character.

Multi-gender attraction: Some people who are attracted to many genders describe themselves as bisexual, others as pansexual, and still others describe themselves differently. People who experience multi-gender attraction may have a vibrant spectrum of kink partners to play with.

Munch: Originally called "burger munches," these social events provide opportunities for kinky people to meet in a casual context for networking, most often with food.

Nesting Partner: A partner you live with and make a home with, regardless of whether they are a sexual or kink partner.

Neurodivergent: Being neurodivergent (or neuro*atypical*) is a spectrum of experience where a person's brain processes information differently from other (neuro*typical*) people. This category includes but isn't limited to people with autism, attention deficit and hyperactivity (ADHD), and giftedness.

Nipple clamps: Kink equipment used to maintain pressure on the nipples for pleasure.

Non-monogamy: A relationship configuration wherein partners agree that sexual and/or romantic activity is not exclusive to two partners, and that passing, romantic, or even deep abiding relationships outside the couple are welcome.

Object insertion: Penetration of a partner by anything other than a body part.

Orgasm: A sometimes-culminating event of sexual arousal and pleasure, that may or may not involve ejaculation, and often involves intense physical contractions of the testicles, penis, vagina, and uterus. Orgasms are not a must for achieving intense kink or sexual pleasure. Kinksters often pursue a wide variety of "ultimate" pleasure sources, including but not limited to orgasm.

Orgasm control: Exerting power over one or more partner's orgasms, including when and if they happen at all.

Orgasm denial: When one person in a scene doesn't allow another to climax.

Paddling: Spanking with tools, particularly with a broad flat surface.

Pain play: Pursuit or infliction of any kind of pain in a kink scene for pleasure.

Parasocial relationship: A relationship with a celebrity, person on social media, or fictional character, wherein the person following the celebrity or character develops a feeling of intimacy and meaning in the relationship.

Pegging: When a person wears a strap-on to augment the size of their flesh genitals in order to penetrate someone, particularly when a women does so to a man.

Pet play: Role-play in which one or more partner pretends to be a pet; cat and dog pet play are by far the most common forms.

Pig play: Getting as down and dirty with another kinkster as arises in the moment. This doesn't involve being an actual pig, but refers to the greediness of the players.

Play: Kinksters use the word "play" to refer to expressing or practicing their kinks.

Play partners: Anyone you engage in kink with, sometimes used to describe people you're not in a formal relationship or romantically involved with.

Polyamory: A relationship of more than two partners built upon consent among relative equals, full disclosure among all partners, and mutual respect, even if each partner has a different role, significance, or meaning in one's life.

Pony play: Role-play involving one or more kinksters taking on the role of a horse or pony. Sometimes this includes bits or bite sticks and other props or costume. Pony play often revolves around the release of not carrying the burden of human responsibility.

Pornography: Sometimes abbreviated "porno," pornography consists of stories, videos, or other media that present sexual acts and scenes as a vehicle of arousal and that may sometimes be incorporated into kink play.

Power play: Sexual activities wherein one or more participants consensually relinquish power to another, and one or more partners assume control, or dominate a sexual situation or relationship, to the delight of all.

Practical sex ed: Kink role-play involving hands-on teaching about sex.

Praise kink: Deriving kink gratification from being complimented or highly praised.

Public use: Consenting in advance to one or more people having free reign to have sex with you wherever and whenever they want, without checking in with you in the moment.

Puppy play: Role-play involving one or more kinkster taking on the role of a puppy. Sometimes this involves wearing a pup hood or tail.

Quirt: A braided riding whip taken from equestrian culture and commonly used in kink.

Rape play: See Consensual non-consent.

Relationship escalator: A typical relationship escalator looks something like this: crushing > dating > kissing and making out > having sex > becoming sexually exclusive > dating over time > moving in together > becoming engaged > getting married. The classic relationship escalator creates a direct link between escalating, exclusive emotional and sexual involvement, and monogamous, lifelong commitment.

Restraints: Anything that limits mobility for the purposes of pleasure. For example, a straight-jacket or handcuffs.

Restrictions: Constraining expression, activities, or body movement in a scene or on an ongoing basis may be a form of kink.

Rimming: Licking or sucking the rim of the anus for pleasure.

Role: In the world of kink, the word "role" can refer to Doms, subs, and switches, or it can refer to a more specific character that a kinkster takes on during role-play, like the role of a doctor.

Role-play: Kink play involving fantasy situations or world-building and/or taking on characters.

Rubber: Rubber is among the most prominent of material fetishes; kinksters love the specific texture and feeling of restraint that rubber provides.

Safety: While co-creating scenes, talk often centers around safety, both physical and emotional. But physical and emotional safety are embedded in society as a whole, so that people in the scene may possess very different *foundations* of safety based on race, gender, ability, citizenship, age, and so on. Scene agreements can't guarantee emotional or physical safety, but they can account for and address inequities while attempting to create a container for emotional risk, sexual experimentation, and meaningful care.

Safeword: The emergency brakes on a kink scene: a term or signal that partners agreed on ahead of time that they will use if they need things to stop for any reason.

Saint Andrew's Cross: Kink equipment shaped like a large letter X that a person can be bound to in order to receive impact play.

Scat: A synonym for human excrement or sh*t and also the preferred term for kinksters who pursue this kind of play.

Scene: The co-created, often choreographed, and yet anarchic arena of kink play.

Scene container: The construct for a kink scene wherein limits are set and activities may be painstakingly discussed and outlined in advance.

Service: When a kinkster is emotionally or sexually gratified by acts of service, they are often called a service-bottom. Acts of service can include a wide array of activities, from doing your Top's laundry, to walking their dog, to being available for specific kink practices or sexual acts.

Sex jail: A stifling enclosure that is constructed when one partner non-consensually imposes the terms of appropriate or acceptable desires or sexual activities in a fleeting or ongoing sexual partnership. In this case, one person's desires rule and the other is jailed.

Sex machines: Kinetic devices used for repeated penetration.

Sexphobia: See "Anti-sex or sex-negative culture."

Sexology: The historic and current study of sex. Polish-Jewish researcher Magnus Hirschfeld is often referred to as its founder.

Sex swing: A harness used to suspend one partner during sex; swings can create better access for kink activities or penetration and can hold or even partly immobilize a scene partner.

Sexually Transmitted Infection (STI): Any infection that is passed from one person to another during sex. It is an updated term for sexually-transmitted diseases (STDs).

Shame: The feeling or belief a person holds that they are inappropriate, wrong, or broken. Sometimes brought on by a specific or historic act of abuse or a mistake. Kinksters often play with shame, pressing on feelings of humiliation or degradation as a multiplier for their arousal.

Shibari: A Japanese rope bonding practice, with single and double column ties providing a gateway into a complex and compelling aesthetic world of ties. In Japan, it is called *kinbaku* (緊縛), which literally translates as "tight binding,"

Sixty-nine: Two partners simultaneously performing oral sex on one another by flipping their bodies for parallel access. The two entwined bodies are said to resemble the numerals six and nine.

Sleep play: Kink where partners agree in advance that one person can initiate sex or a kink activity while the other is sleeping. This can also be role-played.

Sleep sacks: See Bags.

Sling: A sex swing attached to hooks or a set of bars that allows it to stand on its own.

Small Penis Humiliation (SPH): Verbal humiliation centered on penis size. This can be based in the reality of a person's body or it can be a form of role-play regardless of actual genital size.

Solo poly: You're the hub of your poly life. Your hub may have zero or many relationship spokes on its wheel. Often, solo poly people live solo and have no *relationship escalator* in their partnerships.

Somatic practices: Mind-body techniques to ground yourself, cultivate calm, and relieve stress and pain.

Sounding: Insertion of thin objects into the urethra for pleasure.

Spit roast: A sexual formation of three people in which one is being penetrated by the other two simultaneously but at opposite ends.

Spreader bars: Kink gear made up of a bar with cuffs for the ankles or wrists on either end so that the wearer is forced to keep them apart.

Steampunk: A genre of science-fiction using the symbols of 19th century industrialization in futuristic ways. This gave birth to a world of fashion and style that can be used as a part of costume play in kink settings.

Strap-on: A dildo designed to be worn over the groin or pubic mound so that it can be used to stimulate or penetrate a partner.

Stripping/disrobing: Removing clothing to stimulate others.

Submission: A kink for surrendering power to a partner.

Submissive (sub): The person who takes the submissive role in a kink scene or the one who surrenders power in the kink dynamic (see Chapter 4).

Surveillance: A kink for consensually monitoring someone or being monitored in any realm of life, such as eating, spending, movements, or even relationships, for pleasure.

Suspension: A form of bondage in which someone is strung up from overhead.

Teasing: Kink play in which something is implied to be coming, such as an orgasm, but it is pulled back and denied before that promise is actually fulfilled.

Tentacles: A role-play kink coming from pornographic images and stories of tentacled creatures using their limbs to simultaneously restrain or engulf someone and penetrate them.

Top: Top has two meanings in the kink world. Sometimes it is used as a synonym for Dom or Dominant in a Dom/sub pairing. When it comes to penetrative sex, it can also mean the partner doing the penetrating. These two meanings may not always line up. For example, a bottom (the partner being penetrated) could be the Dom in charge of the scene.

Transformation: A kink for the idea of changing your physical form or the way you present, such as transforming your style, gender, or human presentation including being forced to make this change.

Transparency: In kink world this means that every partner in a scene is fully informed about all the intimate relationships in the mix and about all the crucial health conditions, needs and limits that are operating.

Trigger: A word, action, gesture, sight, sound, or smell that moves you from the present moment to a previous moment that involved harm or violation.

Unicorn: A rare find in sex or kink worlds, hence the moniker — because unicorns don't exist in real life. In the past, unicorn was often used to refer to a mythical bisexual woman sought after by couples for play or romance, who had few needs herself, or a desire for attachment.

Uniform: A kink that references clothing worn as a uniform in real life, including military or police uniforms, school uniforms, or a professional uniform, such as a nurse's uniform or doctor's lab coat.

Verse (or versatile): Describes being interested in Topping and bottoming sexually, which may involve penetrating one's partner anally or vaginally, or being receptive to penetration, depending on a partner's interests.

Vibrators: A vibrating toy used for sexual stimulation of yourself or partners; sometimes inserted, or pressed against sensitive sex parts, like a nipple or clitoris.

Virgin: Someone who is "new" to sex. This term is often used to categorize someone who has not had penetrative sex. However, this construction of "virgin" claims penetrative sex as the ultimate act, or the only "real" sex, which is a patriarchal and discredited idea. Kinksters like to create scenes around sexual novices or naivete for pleasure.

Voyeurism: A kink for watching others display their bodies, engage in kink play, or have sex.

War symbolism: Using references to warfare or specific historical wars in kink clothing or play.

Watersports: Peeing on a scene partner's body or into the mouth during kink play, also known as piss play.

Whipping: Some kinksters enjoy hitting or being hit by their partners with various kinds of implements including floggers and bullwhips.

Yellow light: Used by some in kink play as a verbal signal to their partner(s) that they are approaching but have not yet reached their limit.

Resources

Please note: Some of these offerings are in the realm of fantasy and thus do not center mutual respect and consent.

Movies

>> *Belle du Jour,* dir. Luis Buñuel (1967)

>> *The Bitter Tears of Petra Von Kant,* dir. Rainer Werner Fassbinder (1972)

>> *The Night Porter*, dir. Liliana Cavani (1974)

>> *Maitresse,* dir. Barbet Schroder (1975)

>> *Jeanne Dielman, 23 Quai du Commerce, 1080 Bruxelles,* dir. Chantal Ackerman (1976)

>> *Cruising,* dir. William Friedkin (1980)

>> *Seduction: The Cruel Woman*, dirs. Monika Truet and Elfi Mikesch (1985)

>> *9½ Weeks,* dir. Adrian Lyne (1986)

>> *Sex, Lies, and Videotape*, dir. Steven Soderbergh (1989)

>> *A New Love in Tokyo* (愛の新世界), dir. Banmei Takahashi (1994)

>> *Total Eclipse*, dir. Agnieszka Holland (1995)

>> *Bound*, dirs. The Wachowskis (1996)

>> *Crash*, dir. David Cronenberg (1996)

>> *East Palace, West Palace* (东宫西宫), dir. Zhang Yuan (1996)

>> *Sick: The Life and Death of Bob Flanagan, Supermasochist,* dir. Dick Kirby (1997)

>> *The Piano Teacher*, dir. Michael Haneke (2001)

>> *Secretary*, dir. Steven Shainberg (2002)

>> *Swimming Pool*, dir. François Ozon (2003)

>> *A Dirty Shame*, dir. John Waters (2004)

>> *Shortbus*, dir. John Cameron Mitchell (2006)

>> *Lust, Caution* (色, 戒), dir. Ang Lee (2007)

>> *Spider Lilies* (刺青), dir. Zero Chou (2007)

>> *Tied*, Hélène Fillières (2013)

>> *The Ceremony*, dir. Lina Mannheimer (2014)

>> *Duke of Burgundy*, dir. Peter Strickland (2014)

>> *Elle*, dir. Paul Verhoeven (2016)

>> *The Handmaiden* (아가씨), dir. Park Chan-wook (2016)

>> *Phantom Thread*, dir. Paul Thomas Anderson (2017)

>> *Professor Marson and the Wonder Woman*, dir. Angela Robinson (2017)

>> *Mapplethorpe*, dir. Ondi Timoner (2018)

>> *Dogs Don't Wear Pants*, dir. J-P Valkeapää (2019)

>> *Liberté*, dir. Albert Serra (2019)

>> *Love and Leashes* (모럴센스), dir. Park Hyun-jin (2022)

>> *Babygirl*, dir. Halina Reijn (2024)

>> *Pillion*, dir. Harry Lighton (2025)

Television

>> *Real Sex* (1990–2009)

>> *London Spy* (2015)

>> *BONDiNG* (2019–2021)

>> *Sex Education* (2019–2023)

>> *Sex, Love, & Goop* (2021)

>> *Dying for Sex* (2025)

Podcasts

>> *Dying for Sex* with Molly Kochan & Nikki Boyer, https://wondery.com/shows/dying-for-sex/

>> *Just Sex: Mapping Your Desire* with Jaime M. Grant, www.justsexpodcast.com

>> *Kinky, Nerdy, and Poly* with G & M, https://knppodcast.com

>> *Love in a F*cked Up World* with Dean Spade, www.deanspade.net/podcast

>> *Making Polyamory Work* with Libby Sinback, www.makingpolyamorywork.com

>> *Savagelovecast* with Dan Savage, https://savage.love/lovecast

>> *Sloppy Seconds* with Big Dipper & Meatball, https://foreverdogpodcasts.com/podcasts/sloppy-seconds/

>> *Why are People Into That?!* with Tina Horn, https://pod.link/798960436

Fiction

>> *Acts of Service: A Novel* by Lillian Fishman

>> *All Fours* by Miranda July

>> *Bad Behavior* by Mary Gaitskill

>> *Consumed* by David Cronenberg

- >> *Crash* by J.G. Ballard

- >> *Doing It for Daddy: Short and Sexy Fiction about a Very Forbidden Fantasy,* ed. Patrick Califia

- >> *For Real* by Alexis Hall

- >> "Gospodar," by Garth Greenwell, (short story)

- >> *Kink: Stories*, eds. R.O. Kwon and Garth Greenwell

- >> *Leash* by Jane DeLynn

- >> *The Leather Daddy and the Femme: an erotic novel in several scenes and a few conversations* by Carol Queen

- >> *Lost Boi* by Sassafras Lowrey

- >> *Luster* by Raven Leilan

- >> *Macho Sluts: Erotic Fiction*, ed. Patrick Califia

- >> *The Marketplace Series* by Laura Antoniou

- >> *New Animal* by Ella Baxter

- >> *Return to Nevèrÿon* by Samuel Delaney

- >> "Safeword" by R.O. Kwon (short story)

- >> *Telepaths Don't Need Safewords* by Cecilia Tan

- >> *Trash: Short Stories* by Dorothy Allison

- >> *Venus in Fur* by David Ives (play)

Nonfiction and Memoir

- >> "BDSM and Race Play," by Mollena Williams-Haas (essay)

- >> *Coming To Power: Writing and Graphics on Lesbian S/M*, ed. Samois

- >> *The Diary of Anaïs Nin* by Anais Nin

- >> *The Ethical Slut: A Practical Guide to Polyamory, Open Relationships, and Other Freedoms in Sex and Love* by Janet W. Hardy and Dossie Easton

- >> *A Guide to the Alternative Swinging Lifestyle* by Trixy Jinx

- >> *In the Dream House* by Carmen Maria Machado

- >> *Kink on a Budget: Guide to Affordable & Quality DIY Kinky Toys* by Alexander Mind and Lorelei Steel

>> *Love in a F*cked Up World: How to Build Relationships, Hook-Up, and Raise Hell Together* by Dean Spade

>> *My Dangerous Desires: A Queer Girl Dreaming Her Way Home* by Amber Hollibaugh

>> *The New Bottoming Book* by Dossie Easton and Janet W. Hardy

>> *The New Topping Book* by Dossie Easton and Janet W. Hardy

>> *Playing Well with Others: Your Field Guide to Discovering, Exploring and Navigating the Kink, Leather, and BDSM Communities Paperback* by Lee Harrington and Mollena Williams

>> *Pleasure Activism: The Politics of Feeling* Good by adrienne maree brown

>> *Polyamory For Dummies* by Jaime M. Grant

>> *Screw the Roses, Send Me the Thorns: The Romance and Sexual Sorcery of Sadomasochism* by Molly Devon and Philip Miller

>> *Seductive Art of Japanese Bondage* by Midori

>> *Serve: Diary of an Old Guard Slave* by V. M. Johnson

>> *THE Sex & Pleasure Book: Good Vibrations Guide to Great Sex for Everyone* by Carol Queen and Shar Rednour

>> *Susie Sexpert's Lesbian Sex World* by Susie Bright

>> *Ties that Bind: SM / Leather / Fetish / Erotic Style: Issues, Commentaries and Advice* by Guy Baldwin

>> *Transland: Consent, Kink & Pleasure* by Mx. Sly

>> "Uses of the Erotic: The Erotic as Power" by Audre Lorde (essay)

>> *Whip Smart, A Memoir* by Melissa Febos

>> *Woof!: Perspectives Into The Erotic Care & Training of The Human Dog* by Michael Daniels

Kinky Playlist

>> "Blood, Sex, and Booze" by Green Day

>> "Closer" by Nine Inch Nails

>> "Discipline" by Janet Jackson

>> "Dominated Love Slave" by Green Day

>> "Erotica" by Madonna

>> "Fetish" by Joan Jett

>> "Freak on a Leash" by Korn

>> "Glory Box" by Portishead

>> "Hey Pretty" by Poe

>> "I Like it Rough" by Lady Gaga

>> "In the Modern World" by Fontaines DC

>> "It's Amazing to Be Young" by Fontaines DC

>> "Justify My Love" by Madonna

>> "Master and Servant" by Depeche Mode

>> "My Kink is My Karma" by Chappell Roan

>> "Pleasure Slave" by Manowar

>> "S&M" by Rihanna

>> "Sucia" by Kehlani

>> "Superfreak" by Rick James

>> "Teeth" by Lady Gaga

>> "Use Me Up" by Bill Withers

>> "Venus in Furs" by Velvet Underground

Apps and Resource Sites

>> **Feeld** (`https://feeld.co`). Kink-inclusive app for all genders and sexualities.

>> **FetLife** (`https://fetlife.com`). Kink-specific site for all genders and sexualities, particularly useful for the local event listings calendar.

>> **Recon** (`www.recon.com`). Kink-specific app centered on gay and bi men.

Advocacy and Support Organizations

>> **Accountable Communities Consortium,** Shannon Perez-Darby, `https://accountablecommunities.com`

>> **Chosen Family Law Center,** `https://chosenfamilylawcenter.org`

- **» Eulenspiegel Society (TES),** `www.tes.org`

- **» Leather Archives & Museum,** `https://leatherarchives.org`

- **» National Association on Mental Illness support groups (NAMI),** `www.nami.org/Support-Education/Support-Groups`

- **» National Coalition for Sexual Freedom (NCSF),** `https://ncsfreedom.org`

- **» National Queer and Trans Therapists of Color Network,** `https://nqttcn.com/`

- **» Society of Janus,** `https://soj.org`

- **» The Alternative Sexualities Research Alliance,** `www.tashra.org`

- **» The Heal Project,** Ignacio Rivera and Aredvi Azad, `https://heal2end.org/links`

- **» Twelve-step programs,** find a free Alcoholics Anonymous, Narcotics Anonymous, or Co-Dependents Anonymous (CoDA) meeting near you by calling 1-800-662-HELP (4357), `www.aa.org/find-aa` and `https://coda.org/find-a-meeting/online-meetings`

- **» Woodhull Freedom Foundation,** `www.woodhullfoundation.org`

Social Groups

- **» Black Rose,** Washington, DC; an educational and support organization for all genders and sexualities, `https://br.org`

- **» Centaur Motorcycle Club,** Washington, DC; men's group centered on motorcycles and leather, host of the annual Mid-Atlantic Leather Weekend, `https://centaurmc.org`

- **» Chicago Hellfire Club,** Chicago, IL; an example of a gay leather club, `https://hellfire13.net`

- **» Chicago Rope,** Chicago, IL; volunteer-based rope education initiative, `https://chicagoropedotcom.wordpress.com/`

- **» Club X,** San Diego, CA; a pansexual education-focused organization, `www.clubxsd.org`

- **» The Eagle,** gay male-centered leather bars in more than thirty cities around the world have adopted the name The Eagle inspired by the New York City bar, The Eagle's Nest, which is now called The Eagle NYC.

- **>> F.I.S.T.,** Baltimore, MD; a leather/BDSM, service, educational, and social organization centered on women, `www.fistwomen.org`

- **>> Lesbian Sex Mafia,** New York City, NY; `https://lesbiansexmafia.org`

- **>> Munches Private Club,** San Antonio, TX; kink social and educational group for all genders and all sexualities, `https://munches.wildapricot.org`

- **>> ONYX,** BIPOC gay and bi men's club, `www.onyxmen.com`

- **>> ONYX Pearls,** leather club for the empowerment of BIPOC women, including trans women, butches, and femmes, as well as nonbinary, genderqueer, trans masculine people of color, `www.onyxpearlsnyne.com`

- **>> San Francisco Leathermen's Discussion Group (SFLDG),** Northern CA; a LGBTQ leather men's organization that hosts events like The Folsom Street Fair.

- **>> Sanctuary Studios,** Los Angeles, CA; dungeon and kink organization for all genders and all sexualities, `https://sanctuarylax.com`

- **>> Sarasota Dark Temple,** Sarasota, FL; dungeon and kink organization for all genders and sexualities, `www.eastcoastkinkevents.com/dungeons/sarasotadarktemple`

- **>> SigMA,** Washington, DC; a male BDSM, Kink, Fetish organization, `www.sigmadc.org`

Events and Contests

- **>> Beyond Leather,** West Palm Beach, FL; annual educational BDSM kinky fetish event for all genders and sexualities, `www.beyondleather.net`

- **>> Cleveland Leather Annual Weekend (CLAW),** Cleveland, OH; annual gay and bi male-centered leather, fetish, and BDSM convention, `www.clawinfo.org`

- **>> Dark Odyssey,** a series of annual kink gatherings for all genders and all sexualities, `https://darkodyssey.com`

- **>> DESIRE Unchained,** a series of west coast queer women-centered kink events, `https://desireunchained.com`

- **>> DomCon New Orleans,** New Orleans, annual kink events for all genders and sexualities centered on BDSM, `https://domcon.com`

- **>> Exxotica,** annual series of sex conventions for all genders and sexualities, `www.exxxoticaexpo.com/about`

» **Folsom Street Fair,** San Francisco, CA; an annual open-air celebration of kink, leather, and LGBTQ culture held in September at the conclusion of the city's "Leather Pride Week," www.folsomstreet.org

» **Frolicon,** Atlanta, GA; annual convention combining all things kinky with all things geeky, https://frolicon.com

» **International Mr. Leather (IML),** Chicago, IL; annual gay and bi male-centered convention and competition celebrating the leather, kink, fetish, and BDSM communities, also hosting other competitions such as International Mr. Bootblack, www.internationalmrleather.com

» **International Ms. Leather,** Piscataway, NJ; annual queer women-centered convention and competition, www.instagram.com/international.mslbb

» **Kinky Kollege,** Chicago, IL; annual kink education event, https://kinkykollege.com

» **Kinkycon,** an annual conference celebrating the education and exploration of BDSM, polyamory, gender identity, sexuality for people of all genders and sexualities, https://kc.gotomyevent.com

» **Know Other Festival,** Jacumba Hot Springs, annual queer women-centered camping festival dedicated to sexuality, healing, and liberation, www.knowotherfestival.com

» **Leather Leadership Conference,** Los Angeles, CA; annual event to empower kink leaders and educators, www.leatherleadership.net

» **Mid-Atlantic Leather,** Washington, DC; annual gay male-centered convention and contest focused on leather, kink, and BDSM, www.leatherweekend.com

» **MIR – Mr. International Rubber,** the largest annual LGBTQ-centered rubber contest and convention, https://mirubber.com

» **National LGBTQ Task Force's Creating Change Conference Sex Track,** the largest annual LGBTQ activist conference featuring a track of programming concerning sexual liberation, www.thetaskforce.org/creating-change

» **Northwest Leather Celebration,** Sacramento, CA; annual LGBTQ-centered kink and leather convention, www.northwestleathercelebration.com

» **Women of Drummer,** an annual celebration of women's leather, play, and community, www.womenofdrummer.com

» **PoHo No Ho(st) Social,** San Francisco, CA; annual series of events hosted by the San Francisco Leathermen's Discussion Group, www.sfldg.org

» **SELF! SouthEast LeatherFest,** Atlanta, GA; an annual educational, fundraising, and social convention for all genders and all sexualities, https://seleatherfest.com/home

» **Sex Down South,** Atlanta, GA; a Southern, BIPOC, women-led kink-affirming sex and sexuality experience, www.sexdownsouth.com

Resorts

>> **Hedonism II,** Jamaican resort known for kink, swinging, and adventuring

>> **Desire Riviera Maya Resort,** clothing-optional Mexican resort for couples only

Help Surviving Violence or Abuse

Kink communities champion consent and mutual respect. If you're being belittled, controlled, or abused by a partner, check out the following resources.

>> **The Network La Red,** a survivor-led organizing to end partner abuse; 1-800-832-1901. The Network's 24-hour hotline provides confidential emotional support, information, referrals, safety planning, and crisis intervention for polyamorous people who are being abused. You don't have to leave or want to leave your relationship to get support, and it's free.

>> **National Sexual Assault Telephone Hotline,** for an emergency call-in number for confidential help with issues surrounding sexual assault, call 1-800-656-4673, https://rainn.org/about-national-sexual-assault-telephone-hotline

These books and videos may also support your healing from interpersonal violence:

>> *Beyond Survival*, eds. Ejeris Dixon and Leah Lakshmi Piepzna-Samarasinha (2020)

>> *The Revolution Starts at Home*, eds. Ching-In Chen, Jai Dulani, and Leah Lakshmi Piepzna-Samarasinha (2016)

>> *What it Takes to Heal: How Transforming Ourselves Can Change the World,* Prentis Hemphill (2024)

>> *Barnard Center for Research on Women's Accountable Communities series,* https://bcrw.barnard.edu/building-accountable-communities/

Index

D

G

H

I

About the Authors

Jaime M. Grant, PhD, author of *Great Sex: Mapping Your Desire*, is an Irish-American sexpert, grassroots researcher, and activist who has been engaged in LGBTQ+, women's, and racial justice movements since the late '80s. Having survived sexist violence and anti-lesbian disownment as a youth, she became a go-to resource on gender and sex as a matter of survival.

This led to doctoral study in gender and sexuality and the creation of the Desire Mapping process, which she has offered for 20 years via individual coaching as well as in workshops at community centers and universities throughout the United States and human rights convenings around the globe — including Russia, China, South Korea, Vietnam, the Philippines, Cyprus, Kenya, South Africa, New Zealand, and Mauritius.

In the '10s, she served as principal investigator for the National LGBTQ Task Force's groundbreaking reports on aging, *Outing Age* (2010) and anti-transgender discrimination, *Injustice at Every Turn: A Report of the National Transgender Discrimination Survey* (2011). In 2017, she co-edited a global anthology on friendship as fuel for movement-building entitled *Friendship as Social Justice Activism*. Most recently, she authored *Polyamory For Dummies* (2024) and co-authored the report of the nation's largest grassroots survey of LGBTQ+ women who partner with women, *"We Never Give up the Fight": A Report of the National LGBTQ+ Women's Community Survey* (2023).

Jack Harrison-Quintana, M.A., is a queer Latino activist, author, and researcher. His work at the intersection of digital advocacy and LGBTQ+ justice has earned him recognition as one of *Foreign Policy* magazine's top geopolitical thinkers of 2016 as well as *Fast Company*'s most creative people in business.

Over the course of his career, Jack has worked with the National LGBTQ Task Force, the National Center for Transgender Equality (NCTE), the Global Trans Research and Advocacy Project (GTRAP), Grindr for Equality, and Khemara, as well as five state and local LGBTQ-related ballot measure campaigns.

Jack has spoken on sexual liberation, as well LGBTQ+ health and safety in over a quarter of the world's countries. He has presented to the National HIV Prevention Conference, International AIDS Conference, ILGA World, and Creating Change. He's also briefed the U.S. House of Representatives; the U.S. Senate; the United Nations; and members of the British Parliament, the Norwegian Stortinget, and the Hong Kong Legislative Council.

Dedications

To the queer kinksters in my life who have given me my world: Dorothy Allison, Naria Lei B. Jordan, M'Bwende Anderson, Amelie Zurn-Galinsky, Jack Harrison-Quintana, Ignacio Rivera, and especially Eric Rofes, whose talk with Suzanne Pharr at Creating Change 1989 helped me leave the kink closet forever. Rest in Power, King. Your kinky brilliance still moves and inspires me. —**Jaime M. Grant**

To the LGBTQ+ and Sexual Liberation movements that have given my life meaning, including everyone in the community of Desire Mappers committed to changing ourselves and changing the world to be more just and more pleasurable. Also, to my Leather Father, David Feaster, and my best friend, Jaime Grant, whose partnership has made this book possible and enabled me to have the life I want. —**Jack Harrison-Quintana**

Authors' Acknowledgments

Special thanks to our two technical editors — Ignacio G. Hutía Xeiti Rivera and Naria Lei B. Jordan — whose contributions amplified and refined so many elements of *Kink For Dummies*, making it a much better book.

Thanks to the intellectual/activist trailblazers who made this work possible, especially Audre Lorde, Essex Hemphill, John D'Emilio, Susan Stryker, Sylvia Rivera and Marsha P. Johnson, Cary Alan Johnson, and Tourmaline.

Thanks to our funder/champion Weston Milliken at the Freeman Foundation and his co-conspirator, Ben Francisco Maulbeck. Thanks to Elizabeth Scott for funding travel so that we can continue to do this work in community.

Thank you to Aaron Hans, our long-time collaborator who came through with a crucial last-minute technological save on this project.

And massive thanks to our team of sexy resistors and collaborators: A., Amelie, Anna, Aredvi, Asha, Bishop, Dean, Elizabeth, E.T., Gina, Ignacio, JD, Kamilah, Mallory, M'Bwende, Mija, Naria, Robin, Romeo, Rox, Shaan, Tia, and Ting Ting. Here's a bit more about them:

>> **A.** Contributions to the book are sometimes anonymous to preserve privacy or safety.

>> **Amelie Zurn-Galinsky** (she series) is a queer polyamorous dyke. She plays as a kinky service switch and works as an organizer, healer, and mother who creates justice in our world for all human bodies, sexualities, and genders. E-mail: azurn2@icloud.com.

- **Anna Meyer** is a mixed-race queer organizer, healing practitioner, and consultant working for social justice and liberation; www.formation healingarts.com.

- **Mx. Aredvi Azad** is a national speaker, trainer, and strategist building the movement for sexual liberation through healing-centered intersectional approaches. They are an Irani-American immigrant and practitioner of transformative relationships living in rural Massachusetts; https://aredviazad.com.

- **Asha Leong** is a life coach, sexual liberator, and writer living in Atlanta; www.dreamingdesires.com.

- **Bishop Howard** LCSW (they/them) is a Black, queer, nonbinary therapist, and sexual liberation activist; www.psychologytoday.com/profile/932330.

- **Dean Spade** is an organizer/writer focused on queer and trans liberation and ending cops, borders, prisons, and U.S. militarism. He is the author of *Love in a F'ed Up World: How to Build Relationships, Hook Up and Raise Hell, Together;* www.deanspade.net.

- **Elizabeth Scott** is a queer, poly dyke living and loving in Minneapolis. @elizscottmpls on Instagram.

- **E.T.** is a genderqueer bi+ switch, tree-kisser, writer, audio artist, and therapist; www.psychologytoday.com/us/therapists/et-townsend-grand-rapids-mi/890532.

- **Gina Mostafa** is the founder and director of the connection/education initiative Queering Existentialism. They are also an educator with sex positive community SUCIA (@sucianyc). Learn more at @queering_existentialism.

- **Ignacio G. Hutía Xeiti Rivera** is a queer, genderfluid, independent-polyamorist healer, activist, and writer; http://beacons.ai/blkbrownred.

- **JD Davids** is a queer, trans, chronically-ill, disabled strategist and writer: The Cranky Queer Guide to Chronic Illness; https://thecrankyqueer.substack.com.

- **Kamilah Glover** is an oral femme, Domme, poly, vampire, healer, and teacher; https://afam.vcu.edu/directory/faculty-affiliates/glover.html.

- **Mallory Sinn** (she/they) is the pen name of a trans feminist scholar and activist who also happens to be a nonbinary trans woman, polyamorous bisexual lesbian, and kinky switch. She can be found on mastodon at https://hachyderm.io/@mallory_sinn.

- **M'Bwende Anderson** is a Black queer sapiosexual butch daddy, motivated by curious minds, principled actions, adventurous spirits, and connected hearts. A nomadic, artsy, book nerd, I love nothing more than family, and playing outside; https://taplink.cc/mbwende.anderson.

» **Mija** (they/two spirit) is an Indigiqueer educator and organizer.

» **Naria Lei B. Jordan** is a radical poly GenderQueer Leather Daddy of Color. Queer BDSM elder (40+ years). DESIRE 2.0 co-owner/producer. Leather title holder. Writer. Queer sex educator. Organizer. Unapologetic rabble-rouser; `https://www.facebook.com/narialei.jordan?mibextid=ZbWKwL`.

» **Robin Nussbaum** is a white, queer, genderqueer advocate for sexual liberation and self-determination for all; `https://linktr.ee/robinnussbaum`.

» **Romeo Jackson** is a Black queer femme scholar-healer-organizer; `https://www.linkedin.com/in/romeojackson/`.

» **Rox Anderson** is a Black, queer, gender nonconforming, multiracial, artivist, kinky, leather top daddy; `http://www.linkedin.com/in/roxanneanderson1`.

» **Shaan Lashun** (he/they) is a Black Leathermxn creating spaces and resources that uplift sex workers, kinksters, and queer and trans people of color. Find Shaan posting about this and that on Facebook or Instagram: @shaanlashun.

» **tia marie** (she/her) is a super Black, queer writer, organizer and co-founder of Sex Down South; @sexdownsouth.

» **Ting Ting Wei (韦婷婷)** is a queer and feminist activist, a feminist therapist and supervisor based in southern China. She makes documentaries and conducts research on gender and queer issues.

Publisher's Acknowledgments

Acquisitions Editor: Alicia Sparrow

Project Editor: Donna Wright

Technical Editors: Ignacio Rivera and Naria Lei B. Jordan

Senior Managing Editor: Kristie Pyles

Production Editor: Magesh Elangovan

Cover Image: © AlxCreate/stock.adobe.com